The Nurse

at

Allergology and Immunology

The complete Guide

ALEXANDRE CAREWELL

Table of contents

« Allergology and Immunology are a bit like being a detective specialising in the mysteries of the human body. The allergist tracks down what makes you sneeze, itch and blush, while the immunologist coaches the body's defence team, making sure every cell is ready to fight off unwanted invaders. Together, they make sure you don't sneeze too much and that your body shield is always in top form! »

Chapter 1:
INTRODUCTION
ALLERGOLOGY AND IMMUNOLOGY

Definition and role
Allergology and Immunology

Allergology and immunology are two closely related medical disciplines, concerned respectively with the mechanisms of allergic reactions and the functions of the immune system. Their scope is vast, encompassing a wide range of clinical manifestations, from simple seasonal rhinitis to complex immunodeficiencies, and thus affecting a significant proportion of the population.

Allergology is primarily concerned with the way in which our bodies overreact to certain substances, known as allergens. These allergens may be present in our environment, such as pollen, dust or food. Most people can be exposed to these substances without any problem, but for others this exposure triggers an allergic reaction. This hypersensitivity of the immune system can manifest itself in symptoms as mild as sneezing or as severe as anaphylactic shock, a potentially fatal reaction.

Immunology, on the other hand, is devoted to the study of the immune system, the incredible defence machine that protects our bodies against infection. It is a complex network of cells, tissues and organs that work together to detect and neutralise pathogens such as bacteria, viruses and other threats. However, when this system doesn't work properly, whether it's overactive or underactive, it can give rise to a range of illnesses, from allergies to immunodeficiencies.

The role of Allergology and Immunology is therefore twofold. On the one hand, it involves identifying, diagnosing and treating allergies, helping patients to understand their triggers and to manage or avoid exposure. On the other hand, the speciality seeks to understand dysfunctions in the immune system, whether excessive reactivity or an inability to protect the body, and to implement strategies to correct these anomalies.

Allergology and Immunology are at the crossroads of many medical disciplines, offering a unique understanding of the interaction between our bodies and the environment around us. By navigating this fascinating world of reactions and defences, specialists in these fields play an essential role in ensuring that our immune system functions harmoniously, protecting our health without attacking ourselves.

The importance of specialisation in modern medicine

Modern medicine, with its technological and scientific advances, is at the cutting edge of understanding the human body. At the heart of this understanding lies Allergology and Immunology, a speciality that sheds light not only on the mechanisms by which our body defends itself, but also on how and why it overreacts to substances that are harmless to the majority.

With allergic diseases on the rise like never before, allergy is more relevant than ever. According to the World Health Organisation, hundreds of millions of people suffer from respiratory allergies, and this number is rising all the time. The reasons for this increase remain a subject of active debate, but factors such as pollution, changes in our lifestyles, diet and even excessive hygiene are all suspected of playing a role. Allergies are not just unpleasant; they can seriously impair quality of life and, in extreme cases, be fatal.

Immunology, meanwhile, is the cornerstone of our understanding of many diseases, from common infections to autoimmune diseases and cancer. With the recent development of targeted therapies, such as immunotherapy for the treatment of cancer, it is clear that manipulating the immune system is an exciting frontier of modern medicine. Furthermore, in a world where emerging and re-emerging diseases are a constant concern, a solid understanding of immunology is essential to developing effective prevention and treatment strategies.

The speciality also plays a crucial role in the field of vaccinations, one of the most transformative medical interventions of our time. As debates about vaccination continue to stir public opinion, experts in immunology are essential in demystifying the facts, guiding research and ensuring the efficacy and safety of vaccines.

Allergology and Immunology, at the end of the day, are not just another branch of medicine; they are intrinsically linked to how we interact with our wider environment. They inform and are informed by everything from ecology to sociology, from molecular biology to public health. By unravelling the mysteries of the immune system and providing solutions to the challenges posed by allergies, this specialty continues to shape modern medicine, promising exciting and essential advances for human health in the years to come.

Role and responsibilities of the nurse in Allergology and Immunology

In the dynamic and complex medical field of allergy and immunology, the nurse plays a central role. Much more than simply supporting the doctor, they are often the first point of contact for patients, playing a crucial role in assessment, education and overall management.

- **Patient assessment** : When patients present with symptoms of allergy or immunodeficiency, it is often the nurse who carries out the initial assessment. She takes a medical history, carries out preliminary tests and assesses the severity and nature of the symptoms. This initial assessment is essential to guide subsequent treatment.
- **Administering tests**: Allergy nurses are trained to perform skin tests, measure immunoglobulin levels, administer challenge tests and other specialized assessments that help determine the underlying cause of a patient's symptoms.
- **Patient education**: One of the most crucial roles of the nurse is to educate patients about their condition. She provides information on the nature of allergies or immune disorders, potential triggers, how to prevent exposure and how to manage an allergic reaction or immune crisis.
- **Treatment administration**: Whether administering immunosuppressants, immunoglobulins or allergen injections for immunotherapy, the nurse is often the one who directly manages the treatments. She must be an expert in the technique, while ensuring the patient's safety and comfort.
- **Patient monitoring**: After a treatment has been administered, patients often need to be monitored for possible reactions. The nurse observes vital signs,

symptoms of allergic reactions and any other side effects.

- **Interdisciplinary collaboration**: The allergology and immunology nurse works closely with a multidisciplinary team of allergists, immunologists, dieticians, social workers and other health professionals. This collaboration ensures holistic patient care.
- **Research and updating knowledge**: Medicine is evolving rapidly, and nurses have a responsibility to keep abreast of the latest research, treatments and guidelines in allergology and immunology. They may also play an active role in clinical research.
- **Emotional support**: Faced with a diagnosis of allergy or immune disorder, many patients experience anxiety, frustration or fear. The nurse offers emotional support, listens to patients' concerns and directs them to appropriate resources.
- **Emergency management**: In the event of a severe allergic reaction, such as anaphylactic shock, the nurse must act quickly to administer emergency treatment and stabilise the patient.

Allergy and Immunology Nurses are educators, therapists, researchers and advocates. Her unique position at the crossroads of clinical care, education and research makes her an indispensable pillar in the care of patients with allergies and immune disorders.

Chapter 2:
ANATOMY AND PHYSIOLOGY
THE IMMUNE SYSTEM

Key components of the immune system

The immune system is a complex, interconnected network of cells, tissues, organs and molecules that work together to defend the body against pathogens and other foreign threats. Its ability to distinguish self from non-self is a marvel of biology, and it relies on several key components to perform its protective functions.

- Immune cells :
  - **Lymphocytes** : These are essential for the adaptive immune response. The main types are T lymphocytes (which can kill infected cells directly or help other immune cells) and B lymphocytes (which produce antibodies).
  - **Phagocytes** : These cells "eat" the invaders. The macrophage is a well-known phagocyte, as is the neutrophil.
  - **NK (Natural Killer) cells**: These are capable of directly killing certain infected or tumour cells.
- **Antibodies**: These are special proteins produced by B lymphocytes in response to a specific antigen. They bind to this antigen, marking it for destruction or directly neutralising its function.
- Lymphoid organs :
  - **Bone marrow**: This is the birthplace of blood cells, including most immune cells.

- **The thymus**: This is where the T lymphocytes mature.
- **Lymph nodes**: These act as filters, capturing pathogens and exposing them to immune cells.
- **The spleen**: This filters the blood, exposing it to immune cells and destroying old red blood cells.
- Physical and chemical barriers :
  - **The skin**: This is the first line of defence, acting as a physical barrier.
  - **Mucous membranes**: found in the respiratory, digestive and genitourinary tracts, they secrete mucus which traps pathogens.
  - **Digestive enzymes**: In the stomach, they destroy many pathogens that are ingested.
- **Cytokines and chemokines**: These are signalling proteins which modulate the activity of the immune system, promoting or inhibiting various responses.
- **The complement system**: This is a set of blood proteins which, when activated, can perforate the membrane of bacteria and destroy them.
- **Dendritic cells**: These "present" fragments of pathogens to T lymphocytes, playing an essential role in linking innate and adaptive immunity.

The coordination of these components enables the immune system to mount a rapid defence against threats (innate immunity) while developing an immune memory for previously encountered threats (adaptive immunity). It is this ability to 'remember' that is exploited when we use vaccines to prevent disease. In the magnificent ballet of immunity, each component plays an essential role in ensuring the health and well-being of the individual.

How it works...
the immune system

The immune system is a marvel of coordination and adaptability. It protects the body against pathogens such as viruses, bacteria and parasites, as well as tumour cells. Its ability to differentiate between what belongs to the body (the self) and what is foreign (the non-self) is fundamental to its function. Here's how it works:

- **Innate immunity**: This is the first line of defence, offering a rapid but non-specific response against invaders.
    - **Physical barriers**: Skin and mucous membranes prevent pathogens from entering.
    - **Inflammatory response**: In the event of injury or infection, dilated blood vessels allow more white blood cells to reach the site, causing redness, heat and swelling.
    - **Phagocytosis**: Phagocytes, like macrophages, "eat" the invaders.
    - **Complement proteins**: These can directly attack the membrane of the pathogen or mark it for phagocytosis.
- **Adaptive immunity**: This takes longer to develop, but is specific and has an immune memory.
    - **T lymphocytes**: Once they have matured in the thymus, they can recognise specific antigens by means of receptors. Some, the cytotoxic T cells, destroy infected cells directly, while the helper T cells stimulate other parts of the immune system.
    - **B lymphocytes**: After activation, they differentiate into plasma cells which produce antibodies specific to an antigen. These

antibodies can neutralise or mark the pathogen for destruction.
- **Immune memory**: After an initial exposure, memory B and T lymphocytes are retained. If the same pathogen is encountered again, the response is faster and stronger.
- Communication and regulation :
  - **Cytokines**: These proteins signal and coordinate activity between different immune cells. They can promote or inhibit an immune response.
  - **Regulatory cells**: Certain cells, such as regulatory T lymphocytes, help to modulate or switch off the immune response to prevent damage to healthy tissue.
- Recognition of self and non-self:
  - **Major histocompatibility complexes (MHC)**: These proteins on the surface of cells display pieces of antigen. MHC class I is present on almost all cells and shows what is "normal". MHC class II is present on certain immune cells and shows foreign antigens.
- Surveillance and defence against cancer:
  - **Anti-tumour immunity**: The immune system recognises and targets abnormal cells. NK cells and cytotoxic T lymphocytes play a particularly important role in recognising and destroying tumour cells.

The immune system is a marvel of balance: too active, and it can attack the body's own tissues, leading to autoimmune diseases; not active enough, and it leaves the body vulnerable to infection. Its proper functioning is therefore essential to our survival.

Imbalances and immune deficiency

The immune system is essential for protecting the body against foreign invaders. However, it can sometimes malfunction, leading to imbalances or failures. These abnormalities can make the individual more vulnerable to infection, trigger reactions against his or her own tissues, or lead to hypersensitivity to generally harmless substances.

- Immunodeficiencies :
    - **Primary immunodeficiencies**: These genetic disorders affect the body's ability to fight infection. Examples: IgA deficiency, X-linked agammaglobulinaemia.
    - **Secondary immunodeficiencies**: These result from other diseases or medical treatments. For example, HIV/AIDS affects T lymphocytes, while chemotherapy or corticosteroid therapy can reduce immune activity.
- Autoimmune diseases :
    - These conditions occur when the immune system mistakenly attacks the body's own cells and tissues. Examples include multiple sclerosis (targeting the nervous system), systemic lupus erythematosus (affecting several organs), or rheumatoid arthritis (targeting the joints).
- Allergies:
    - Allergic reactions occur when the immune system overreacts to a normally harmless substance, called an allergen. This can lead to symptoms such as hives, asthma or, in severe cases, anaphylactic shock.

- Inflammatory disorders :
  - Sometimes the immune system can cause excessive or inappropriate inflammation, even in the absence of infection or injury. Diseases such as Crohn's disease or ulcerative colitis are examples.
- Cancers of the immune system :
  - These cancers, such as leukaemia and lymphoma, originate in the cells of the immune system itself. They can impair immune function and often require aggressive medical intervention.
- Rejection reactions :
  - After an organ transplant, the recipient's immune system may recognise the new organ as foreign and attack it, leading to graft rejection. Immunosuppressants are then prescribed to reduce this reaction.
- Immune activation syndromes :
  - In some cases, excessive and uncontrolled activation of the immune system can occur, leading to severe systemic symptoms. Cytokine release syndrome, sometimes observed after certain immunotherapies, is one example.

These imbalances and failures demonstrate the crucial importance of a well-regulated immune system. Early recognition and appropriate management of these conditions are essential to prevent complications and improve patients' quality of life.

Chapter 3:
THE MAIN ALLERGIC AND IMMUNOLOGICAL DISEASES

Respiratory allergies

Respiratory allergies are among the most common allergic conditions. They result from an exaggerated immune response by the body to allergens in the air we breathe. They can affect the upper respiratory tract, such as the nose, or the lower respiratory tract, such as the bronchi.

- Causes of respiratory allergies :
    - **Pollen**: Pollen grains from trees, grasses and herbs are common allergens.
    - **Dust mites**: These tiny creatures live in household dust and are a major cause of respiratory allergies.
    - **Animal hair**: The proteins present in saliva, urine and animal dander can cause allergic reactions.
    - **Mould**: Mould spores present in damp environments are also potential allergens.
    - **Cockroach**: Droppings and body parts can be allergens for some people.
- Symptoms:
    - **Allergic rhinitis**: sneezing, itchy nose, blocked or runny nose, watery and itchy eyes.
    - **Allergic asthma**: coughing, shortness of breath, wheezing and chest tightness. This is an inflammation of the lower respiratory tract in response to an allergen.

- Diagnosis:
  - **Skin   tests**: Allergen extracts are applied to the skin using a small prick to determine the allergens responsible.
  - **Blood test (specific   IgE)**: Measures the amount of IgE antibodies produced in response to certain allergens.
  - **Peak expiratory flow   measurement**: Used to assess lung function in asthma sufferers.
- Treatments :
  - **Allergen avoidance**: The best way to manage an allergy is to avoid the allergen. For example, by using anti-dust mite covers or limiting exposure to pets.
  - **Symptomatic medication**: Antihistamines, nasal corticosteroids, bronchodilators and others may be prescribed.
  - **Immunotherapy (desensitisation)**: This aims to gradually accustom the body to the allergen in order to reduce the severity of the allergic reaction.
- Prevention :
  - **Environmental control**: Reduce humidity to control mould, use air purifiers, and avoid sleeping with windows open during the pollen season.
  - **Education**: Understanding your own allergy, knowing what triggers it and how to avoid them.

Respiratory allergies, if not properly managed, can significantly affect an individual's quality of life. A multidisciplinary approach, involving allergists, lung specialists and, of course, specialist nurses, is often necessary to ensure optimal treatment.

Food and skin allergies

Food and skin allergies are common manifestations of abnormal immune reactivity to normally harmless substances. They can vary in severity, from mild itching to life-threatening reactions.

- **Food allergies :**
    - Causes:
        - Certain foods are more frequently responsible for allergies, such as peanuts, cow's milk, eggs, fish, shellfish, soya, wheat and nuts.
    - Symptoms:
        - These allergies can cause itchy mouth, swelling of the lips or throat, skin rashes, abdominal pain, diarrhoea, vomiting and, in the most serious cases, anaphylactic shock.
    - Diagnosis:
        - Skin test, blood test to detect specific IgE, and oral provocation test under medical supervision.
    - Treatments:
        - Strict avoidance of the food allergen, antihistamines and epinephrine auto-injectors to treat anaphylactic reactions.

- **Skin allergies:**
- Contact dermatitis:
        - Caused by direct contact with an allergen (e.g. nickel, latex, perfumes, preservatives).
        - Symptoms: redness, itching, blistering.
    - Diagnosis: patch test.
        - Treatment: avoidance of the allergen, corticosteroid creams.

- <u>Hives:</u>
  - Skin eruptions characterised by raised, itchy red patches.
  - Can be triggered by food, medication, insect bites or other factors.
- Diagnosis: history, skin tests, blood tests.
- Treatment: antihistamines, avoidance of triggers.
  - Atopic dermatitis (eczema):
  - Inflammatory skin disease with an allergic component.
- Symptoms: dryness, redness, itching.
- Treatment: intense hydration, corticosteroid creams, avoidance of identified allergens.

- **Prevention and education:**
  - The best strategy for managing allergies is to prevent exposure to identified allergens.
  - Educating patients and those around them is crucial, particularly in terms of recognising the early signs of an allergic reaction and knowing how to intervene, notably through the use of an epinephrine auto-injector.

Both food and skin allergies require careful, individualised care. Nurses play a crucial role in educating and monitoring patients and implementing action plans in the event of an allergic reaction. Close collaboration with allergists and dermatologists ensures optimal care and improved quality of life for patients.

Immune deficiencies primary and secondary

Immune deficiencies represent a heterogeneous group of diseases resulting from a failure of the immune system, which may be due to genetic or acquired factors. These deficiencies can make individuals more susceptible to infections, autoimmune diseases or even cancers.

- **Primary immune deficiency (PID):**
  - Definition:
    - DIPs are hereditary or congenital disorders of the immune system. They are generally diagnosed in childhood, but some may not appear until adulthood.
  - Common types :
    - Congenital agranulocytosis: Neutrophil deficiency.
    - **IgA deficiency**: Lack of immunoglobulin A.
    - **DiGeorge syndrome:** Congenital absence of the thymus.
    - Severe combined immunodeficiency syndrome (SCID): Absence of T and B cell function.
  - Diagnosis:
    - History of infections, blood tests (immunoglobulin assay, lymphocyte count), genetic tests.
  - Treatment :
    - Antibiotic prophylaxis, intravenous or subcutaneous immunoglobulins, bone marrow or stem cell transplants for certain types.
- **Secondary immune deficiency:**
  - Definition:
    - These deficits are not hereditary, but result from an illness or an external condition. They are more common than DIPs.

- Common causes:
  - Diseases (HIV, certain cancers, renal failure), malnutrition, ageing, certain medications (corticosteroids, immunosuppressants), medical treatments (chemotherapy, radiotherapy).
- Diagnosis:
  - Clinical assessment, blood tests, identification of underlying cause.
- Treatment :
  - Targeting the underlying cause (e.g. antiretrovirals for HIV), prophylaxis against infections, immunoglobulins, adjustment of causative drugs.
- **Implications for nursing practice :**
  - Assessment :
    - Nurses need to be aware of the signs and symptoms of recurrent or atypical infections.
  - Education :
    - Inform patients and their families about infection prevention, warning signs and the importance of regular medical check-ups.
  - Treatment management :
    - Administration of immunoglobulins, post-transplant care, management of medication side-effects.
  - Psychological support :
    - Immune deficiencies can have a significant psychological impact, requiring appropriate support.

Understanding immune deficiencies is essential for healthcare professionals. Nurses, in particular, play a key role in the management, education and support of patients living with these deficiencies. Multidisciplinary collaboration with immunologists, haematologists and other specialists is crucial to providing optimal care.

Autoimmune diseases

In the complex world of immunology, autoimmune diseases occupy a special place. They result from an inappropriate attack by the immune system on the body's normal tissues and organs, recognising them as foreign. This dysfunction of the immune system can lead to chronic inflammation and tissue damage.

- Understanding autoimmunity :
    - Definition:
        - Autoimmune diseases develop when the body produces immune responses against its own cells, tissues or organs.
    - Cause:
        - The exact cause remains unknown, but genetic, environmental and hormonal factors appear to play a role.
- Common autoimmune diseases :
    - Rheumatoid arthritis :
        - Affects the joints, causing pain, stiffness and possibly deformity.
    - Systemic lupus erythematosus :
        - Can affect the skin, joints, kidneys, heart and nervous system.
    - Multiple sclerosis :
        - Affects the central nervous system, resulting in impaired mobility, vision and sensation.
    - Type 1 diabetes :
        - Destruction of beta cells in the pancreas, leading to a lack of insulin.

- Hashimoto's disease :
  - Attack on the thyroid gland, often causing hypothyroidism.
- Diagnosis:
  - Based on clinical symptoms, blood tests (for autoimmune antibodies), and sometimes biopsies.
- Treatment :
  - Varies according to the disease, but generally includes immunosuppressants, anti-inflammatories and other treatments specific to the disease.
- Role of the nurse :
  - Assessment :
    - Identify symptoms and potential complications, assess pain and functional impact.
  - Education :
    - Informing patients about their illness, medicines, side-effects and self-care strategies.
  - Treatment management :
    - Administration of medication, monitoring of side effects, care of affected areas.
  - Psychosocial support :
    - Living with an autoimmune disease can be stressful and emotionally difficult. The nurse plays a key role in providing emotional support and counselling.
- Prospects and challenges :
  - Autoimmune diseases can be unpredictable, with periods of flare-up and remission.
  - Current treatments aim to control symptoms and reduce inflammation, but they can have side effects.

- Research continues to explore the underlying causes and develop new, more targeted treatments.

Autoimmune diseases are a vast and complex area of medicine that require in-depth understanding and careful management. The nurse, working with a multidisciplinary team, is at the heart of patient management, providing the care, support and education needed to navigate the challenges of these conditions.

Chapter 4:
DIAGNOSTIC TECHNIQUES
IN ALLERGOLOGY AND IMMUNOLOGY

History and clinical examination

History-taking and clinical examination are the fundamental pillars of medical assessment. In allergy and immunology, these steps are crucial to identifying potential triggers, understanding the nature of reactions and making a precise diagnosis.

- **Case history :**
    - Definition:
        - History-taking is the art of taking a patient's medical history, paying particular attention to symptoms, family history, exposures and any other relevant factors.
    - Importance in Allergology and Immunology :
        - Identification of potential exposures: food, drugs, environment.
    - Chronology of symptoms: onset, duration, severity, and triggering or mitigating factors.
        - Personal and family history: Autoimmune diseases or allergies in the family, vaccinations, frequent infections.
    - Medication and treatment: Use of antihistamines, corticosteroids, episodes of hospitalisation.

- **Clinical examination :**
  - Inspection:
    - Observations of the skin (rashes, urticaria, eczema), eyes (allergic conjunctivitis), nose (rhinitis), mouth and throat.
  - Palpation :
    - Lymph nodes checked, abdominal palpation (to detect any splenomegaly or hepatomegaly).
  - Auscultation :
    - Listening to the lungs to detect wheezing or other abnormalities, heart auscultation.
  - Specific tests :
    - Skin tests to detect allergies, pulmonary function tests and other relevant tests depending on symptoms.
- Role of the nurse :
  - Preparing the patient :
    - Explain the process, reassure the patient, ensure that the patient is in the best possible condition for the examination (for example, having avoided antihistamines before a skin test).
  - Assistance during the exam :
    - Assisting the doctor by preparing and administering tests, observing the patient's reaction and ensuring comfort.
  - Education :
    - Explain the results, instructing the patient on symptom management, medication and preventive measures.
  - Documentation:
    - Take detailed, accurate notes on symptoms, test results and recommendations.

- **Specific challenges and considerations :**
  - The sometimes elusive nature of allergies or immune disorders may require repeated visits and in-depth assessment.
  - Allergic tests can be uncomfortable and require close monitoring for possible reactions.
  - Establishing a relationship of trust is essential to obtaining accurate and complete information.

The history and clinical examination are essential steps in making a diagnosis in allergology and immunology. The nurse plays a central role in this process, liaising between the patient and the doctor, facilitating the examination and providing essential care and education. In this field, every detail counts, and careful assessment can make all the difference to patient care.

Skin tests

In the field of allergology, skin tests play a predominant role in identifying the allergens responsible for a patient's symptoms. Although simple on the surface, these tests require precise expertise and meticulous interpretation.

- Principle of skin tests :
  - Introduction :
    - Skin tests involve exposing the skin to small quantities of potential allergens to see if a reaction occurs.
  - Methodology :
    - Allergens are generally applied to the patient's forearm or back using a small lancet that lightly pricks the skin.

- A positive reaction generally manifests itself as itching, redness or a rise in the skin similar to a mosquito bite.
- Types of skin tests :
  - Prick test :
    - Drops containing allergens are placed on the skin, followed by a gentle prick through the drop.
  - Intradermal test :
    - A small amount of allergen is injected just below the surface of the skin.
  - Patch tests :
    - The allergens are applied in patches which are then fixed to the skin, usually for 24 to 48 hours.
- Role of the nurse :
  - Preparing the patient :
    - Inform the patient about how the test will be carried out, and make sure that the patient has avoided any medications that could interfere with the test, such as antihistamines.
  - Carrying out the test :
    - Apply the allergens carefully and in a specific order, and monitor the patient's reaction during and after the test.
  - Education and advice :
    - Explain the results, advise on the management of identified allergies, and give recommendations for avoiding the allergens in question.
- Interpretation and limitations:
  - A positive reaction indicates that the patient is probably allergic to the allergen tested.
  - However, a positive reaction does not always mean that this allergen is the cause of the patient's symptoms.

- Sometimes there can be false positive or false negative reactions.
- It is crucial to combine the results of skin tests with medical history and other examinations to make an accurate diagnosis.
- Safety precautions :
  - Skin tests are generally safe, but there is a small risk of a serious allergic reaction.
  - The nurse must be trained to recognise and treat any anaphylactic reaction.

Skin testing is an essential tool in the allergist's diagnostic armoury. The nurse, as the central pivot in the process, ensures that the test is carried out correctly, that the patient is well informed, and that safety is maintained at all times. Although this is a routine procedure, its importance in the accurate diagnosis of allergies cannot be underestimated.

Spirometry
and other functional tests

Spirometry, along with other respiratory function tests, is fundamental in the diagnosis and monitoring of lung diseases, particularly those associated with respiratory allergies or immune disorders. These tests assess the capacity of the lungs to inhale and exhale air and are crucial in determining a patient's lung function.

- Spirometry :
  - Definition:
    - Spirometry measures the quantity (volume) and speed (flow) of air that an individual can inhale and exhale.

- Indications:
    - Assessment of symptoms such as dyspnoea, chronic cough or wheezing.
    - Monitoring diseases such as asthma, chronic obstructive pulmonary disease (COPD) and other lung diseases.
    - Assessment of bronchial reactivity.
- Main parameters measured :
    - Forced expiratory volume in seconds (FEV1): volume of air expelled during the first second of forced expiration.
    - Forced Vital Capacity (FVC): total volume of air expelled during forced expiration.
    - The FEV1/FVC ratio, which, if reduced, may indicate obstruction.

- Other functional tests :
    - Bronchial provocation test :
        - Assessment of airway reactivity to different stimuli (such as metacholine).
    - Measurement of peak expiratory flow (PEF) :
        - Measurement of maximum exhalation rate. Useful for monitoring asthma on a daily basis.
    - Plethysmography of the body :
        - Measurement of total lung capacity and residual volume.
- Role of the nurse :
    - Preparing the patient :
        - Explain the process, ensure that the patient has avoided any medication that could interfere with the test, and check that the patient has not had a recent asthma attack.
    - Carrying out the test :
        - Seat the patient, show them how to use the device, guide them through the

test and ensure that the manoeuvres are carried out correctly.
- Interpretation and advice :
  - Read and record the results, discuss the results with the doctor, educate the patient about the meaning of the results and the steps to be taken.
- Precautions and limitations :
  - Tests must be carried out according to strict protocols to guarantee their validity.
  - Patients must be able to perform the manoeuvres correctly, which can be difficult for certain age groups or medical conditions.
  - The tests can cause symptoms in patients with respiratory illnesses, which is why it is so important to have rescue medication available.

Spirometry and other functional tests are essential tools for assessing lung function. The role of the nurse is crucial, not only in carrying out the tests but also in educating and supporting the patient. Properly performed, these tests provide valuable information to guide the diagnosis, treatment and follow-up of lung disorders.

Biological tests

In the world of allergology and immunology, biological tests play a vital role. They enable the underlying immunological mechanisms to be analysed and understood, precise diagnoses to be made, the development of pathologies to be monitored and treatment to be guided. Nurses, who are at the heart of this process, are often the first to make contact with patients, collect the necessary samples and educate them about the significance of these tests.

- Blood samples :
    - Allergy test :
        - Total and specific   IgE assays: to detect sensitisation to specific allergens.
    - Immunoassay :
        - Immunophenotyping: to analyse the different sub-populations of immune cells.
        - Measurement of immunoglobulins (IgA, IgG, IgM, etc.): to assess the humoral immune response.

    - Other analyses :
        - Complete   b l o o d   c o u n t, sedimentation rate, C-reactive protein (CRP): to assess inflammation or other immune system reactions.
- Urine tests :
    - Urinalysis: used to detect kidney abnormalities, often associated with certain autoimmune diseases.
- Skin tests and biopsy :
    - Skin biopsy: in the case of skin lesions, to determine their origin (allergic, autoimmune, other).
- Other samples :
    - Bone marrow puncture, cerebrospinal fluid sampling, biopsies of other organs: as clinically indicated.
- Role of the nurse :
    - Direct debit :
        - Taking blood samples, guiding and reassuring patients, ensuring that samples are properly stored and sent to the laboratory.
    - Education :
        - Inform the patient about the nature and purpose of each test, the expected

results and the procedure for taking samples.
- Advise the patient on any precautions to be taken before the sample is taken (fasting, medication to be avoided, etc.).
- Follow-up:
  - Inform the patient when the results are received, and refer them to the doctor for interpretation and discussion.
- Interpretation and limitations:
  - All results must be interpreted in conjunction with clinical symptoms, medical history and other investigations.
  - Abnormal results do not necessarily mean disease; they often require further tests.
  - Results can be influenced by many factors, including medication, age and other medical conditions.

Biological tests are essential tools in allergology and immunology. Their diversity and specificity provide a unique window on the body's internal mechanisms. The nurse, as the essential link between the patient and the laboratory, plays a pivotal role in carrying out, educating and monitoring these tests, thereby guaranteeing the best possible patient care.

Chapter 5:
A NURSE'S DAILY ROUTINE
IN ALLERGOLOGY AND IMMUNOLOGY

Preparing patients for tests

Proper preparation of patients for allergology and immunology tests is crucial to ensure accurate and reliable results. The nurse is often the first point of contact for the patient and plays a vital role in ensuring that the patient understands the importance of preparation, as well as the specific steps to be followed.

- Patient information and education :
    - Understanding the test :
        - Explain to the patient the nature of the test, its purpose and what it can reveal.
    - Responding to concerns :
    - Answer questions, dispel fears and offer practical advice.
    - Specific instructions :
        - Provide clear instructions on what the patient should do or avoid before the test.
- Preparation for blood sampling :
    - **Fasting**: Some tests require fasting for 8 to 12 hours.
    - **Medication**: Inform the patient of any medications that may interfere with results and discuss the possibility of temporarily discontinuing them.
    - **Emotional and physical state**: Stress or intense exertion may affect certain results.

Advise the patient to relax and avoid intense physical effort before the test.

- Preparation for skin tests :
    - **Antihistamines**: These medicines can distort the results and should often be stopped several days before the test.
    - **Creams and lotions**: Avoid applying topical products to the test area.
    - **Skin condition**: The skin must be in good condition, free from rashes or active lesions.
- Preparation for spirometry :
    - **Bronchodilators**: These may be discontinued before the test, depending on medical advice.
    - **Smoking**: Avoid smoking for at least 6 hours before the test.
    - **Physical effort**: Avoid strenuous exercise before the test.
    - **Hearty meal**: Avoid eating a large meal before the test so as not to restrict lung capacity.
- Preparation for other functional tests :
    - Provide specific guidelines for each test, including dietary restrictions, medicines to be avoided and special physical preparations.
- Reminders and follow-up :
    - **Reminders**: Send reminders by telephone, SMS or e-mail to ensure that the patient remembers the test date and preparation instructions.
    - **Test day**: Before the test begins, briefly review the instructions with the patient and ensure that they have been followed correctly.
    - **After the test**: Inform the patient about what happens next, such as when they can expect to receive the results.

Patient preparation is an essential step in ensuring reliable and accurate test results in allergology and immunology. The nurse, with her patient-centred approach and education and communication skills, is ideally placed to guide the patient through this process.

Administration specific treatments

One of the fundamental tasks of the allergology and immunology nurse is to administer specific treatments. These often complex treatments require special expertise, constant vigilance and excellent communication with the patient to ensure their safety and effectiveness.

- Understanding treatments :
    - **Nature of medicines** : In-depth knowledge of the medicines administered, their mechanisms of action, their benefits and any side-effects.
    - **Specific protocols**: familiarity with administration protocols in terms of dosage, route of administration and frequency.
- Immunomodulating treatments :
    - Allergen immunotherapy (desensitisation) :
        - Preparing and administering doses.
        - Monitor the patient during and after the injection for possible reactions.
        - Patient education on the duration of treatment and the importance of adherence.
    - Biotherapies :
        - Administration of biological drugs, such as monoclonal antibodies.
        - Monitoring potential side-effects and educating patients about what to look out for.

- Treatments for autoimmune diseases :
  - Immunosuppressants :
    - Administration of drugs that reduce the activity of the immune system.
    - Education on how to manage side effects and the importance of following medical recommendations.
  - Corticosteroid therapy :
    - Administration of corticosteroids, with particular attention to dosage and duration of treatment.
    - Make the patient aware of the side effects and the need not to stop treatment abruptly.
- Intravenous administration :
  - Intravenous immunoglobulin (IVIG) :
  - Preparation and administration in accordance with established protocols.
  - Monitoring of potential reactions during infusion.
- Education and follow-up :
  - Clear instructions :
    - Provide the patient with clear instructions on taking medication, monitoring side effects and managing any reactions.
  - Adherence to treatment :
    - Promote the importance of following treatment as prescribed and discuss potential barriers to adherence.
    - Suggest strategies to help patients integrate treatment into their daily routine.
- Communication with the medical team :
  - Working closely with doctors, pharmacists and other healthcare professionals to ensure that the patient receives the optimum

treatment and that any concerns or complications are promptly addressed.

The administration of specific treatments in allergology and immunology is an area in which the nurse plays a crucial role. She is a practitioner, educator and patient advocate, ensuring that each individual receives the safest and most effective care possible.

Therapeutic patient education

Therapeutic education is at the heart of allergy and immunology care. Its aim is to give patients a say in their own health, to provide them with the tools they need to understand their illness and treatment, and to support them in the day-to-day management of their condition. The nurse, thanks to her proximity to the patient and her communication skills, is often at the forefront of this mission.

- Understanding the importance of therapeutic education:
    - **Patient autonomy**: The aim is to enable patients to make informed decisions about their health.
    - **Better adherence to treatment**: A well-informed patient is generally more inclined to follow his or her treatment correctly.
- Assessment of educational needs :
    - **Initial assessment**: Identify the patient's pre-existing knowledge, beliefs and attitudes towards the disease and treatment.
    - **Setting objectives**: Establishing learning objectives tailored to each patient.

- Teaching tools and methods :
    - **Written material**: Brochures, information sheets, monitoring diaries.
    - **Workshops and interactive sessions**: discussion groups, practical workshops, demonstrations.
    - **Digital technologies**: applications, educational videos, online platforms.
- Teaching about illness :
    - **Understanding the disease**: Explanations of the underlying mechanisms, symptoms and prognosis.
    - **Recognising signs and symptoms**: Teaching patients to identify the signs of an exacerbation or allergic reaction.
- Treatment management :
    - **Knowledge of medicines**: Explanation of the different treatments, their modes of action, their benefits and their potential side effects.
    - **Administration of treatment**: Demonstration and training in the correct administration of medication (e.g. use of an inhaler).
- Adopting favourable behaviours :
    - **Allergen avoidance**: Advice on how to avoid patient-specific allergens.
    - **Healthy lifestyle habits**: Encouragement to adopt a healthy lifestyle to improve general health and strengthen the immune system.
- Emergency management :
    - **Personalised action plan**: Development of a plan to manage allergic attacks or exacerbations, including the use of an epinephrine auto-injector.
    - **Recognising the signs of an emergency**: Teaching patients to recognise when they need to seek immediate medical help.

- Evaluation and monitoring :
  - **Regular reassessment**: Regularly check the patient's knowledge, adjust the educational objectives if necessary.
  - **Feedback**: Encouraging patients to share their experiences, challenges and successes.

Therapeutic education is a continuous and collaborative process. The allergology and immunology nurse plays an essential role in ensuring that the patient is informed, supported and confident in the management of their disease, thereby improving both the patient's quality of life and therapeutic outcomes.

Emergency situations: Anaphylaxis and others

Handling emergencies is a crucial aspect of the allergology and immunology nurse's role. These situations require rapid, effective and appropriate intervention to ensure patient safety. Anaphylaxis, in particular, is a major medical emergency that all healthcare professionals must be able to recognise and treat without delay.

- Recognising emergency situations :
  - **Symptoms of anaphylaxis**: Difficulty breathing, swelling of the face or throat, skin rash, fall in blood pressure, disturbance of consciousness.
  - **Other allergic emergencies**: severe asthma, giant urticaria, angioedema without anaphylaxis.

- Intervention in the event of anaphylaxis :
  - **Rapid assessment**: Rapidly assess the patient's condition to determine the severity of the reaction.
  - **Call the emergency services**: In severe cases, contact the emergency services immediately.
  - **Administration of epinephrine**: Use an epinephrine auto-injector as recommended and prescribed by your doctor.
  - **Patient position**: If the patient is conscious, put them in a semi-seated position; if they are unconscious, put them in the lateral safety position.
  - **Continuous monitoring**: Keep a close eye on the patient until help arrives, especially breathing, pulse and blood pressure.
- Other emergency interventions :
  - **Severe asthma**: Administration of bronchodilators, oxygenation if necessary, continuous airway assessment.
  - **Angioedema**: Monitoring of respiratory function, administration of antihistamines or corticosteroids as prescribed.
- Preparation and prevention :
  - **Regular training**: Ensuring ongoing training to keep up to date with emergency protocols and best practice.
  - **Equipment available**: Always have an epinephrine auto-injector, oxygen, bronchodilators and a complete emergency kit at hand.
  - **Patient education**: Teaching patients and their families how to recognise the signs of a severe allergic reaction and how to intervene.

- After the emergency :
  - **Assessment**: Once the situation has stabilised, assess the causes of the reaction and discuss preventive measures.
  - **Medical follow-up**: referring the patient to a specialist for in-depth monitoring and the implementation of a personalised action plan.
  - **Debriefing**: Analysing the situation with the medical team to identify the strengths and any improvements to be made in terms of intervention.

Faced with an emergency situation in allergology and immunology, the nurse must demonstrate a high level of responsiveness and technical skills, as well as providing psychological support to the patient and his or her family. Adequate preparation and regular training are essential to ensure optimal care at these critical moments.

Chapter 6:
PREVENTION
IN ALLERGOLOGY AND IMMUNOLOGY

The importance of allergy prevention

Allergies have become a major public health concern in many countries, due to their growing incidence and potential impact on quality of life. Prevention therefore plays a central role in the strategy for managing this problem. It is an essential component that all healthcare professionals, and allergology nurses in particular, must incorporate into their practice.

- Understanding the epidemiology of allergies :
    - **Increasing prevalence** : Trends in allergy cases over time and in different populations.
    - **Risk factors**: Genetics, environment, lifestyle and other determinants.
- Primary prevention: avoid raising awareness :
    - **Environmental factors**: the importance of air quality and exposure to allergens (pollen, house dust mites, mould, animals, etc.).
    - **Nutrition**: the role of breastfeeding, the introduction of food allergens in infants, diet.
    - **Lifestyle**: Striking a balance between necessary hygiene and overprotection that could be counterproductive.
- Secondary prevention: limiting the progression of the disease :
    - **Early detection**: The importance of early detection for better management and to avoid complications.

- **Allergen avoidance**: avoidance strategies, home layout, choice of materials, advice on limiting exposure.
- **Preventive treatment**: The use of medication or vaccines to prevent symptoms or exacerbations.
- Tertiary prevention: avoiding complications :
  - **Therapeutic education**: training patients to manage their disease, recognise signs of exacerbation and act accordingly.
  - **Regular monitoring**: Regular medical monitoring to adapt treatment and prevent complications.
  - **Management of co-morbidities**: Management of other conditions associated with allergy (asthma, atopic dermatitis, etc.).
- Health promotion and awareness :
  - **Awareness campaigns**: Informing the general public about allergies, their consequences and how to prevent them.
  - **Continuing training**: Ensuring that healthcare professionals keep abreast of the latest advances in allergy prevention.
- Interdisciplinary collaboration :
  - **Networking**: Promoting a collaborative approach with other professionals (GPs, lung specialists, dermatologists, nutritionists, etc.).
  - **Exchanging best practice**: Encouraging professionals to share experiences and preventive strategies.

Prevention is the key to reducing the impact of allergies on individuals and on society as a whole. As front-line healthcare professionals, allergy nurses have a pivotal role to play in implementing preventive strategies, both on an individual level with their patients and on a collective level through their participation in awareness-raising and education initiatives.

Vaccinations:
role, protocols and precautions
for immunocompromised patients

Vaccination is one of the most effective public health interventions, preventing a large number of infectious diseases. However, vaccinating immunocompromised patients poses a number of challenges, as their weakened immune systems may not respond as effectively to the vaccine or may be at greater risk of complications. Nurses play a key role in managing, administering and educating these patients about vaccination.

- Understanding immunodepression :
    - **Definition and causes**: Nature of immunodepression, whether due to disease, treatment or other factors.
    - **Implications for vaccination**: Understanding why vaccine responses may be altered in these patients.
- The role of vaccination in immunocompromised patients :
    - **Enhanced protection**: Despite potentially attenuated responses, vaccination often offers crucial protection against infection for these vulnerable patients.
    - **Herd immunity**: Protect these patients indirectly by vaccinating their family and community.

- Types of vaccines and their indications :
  - **Live attenuated vaccines**: Generally avoided in immunocompromised patients due to the potential risk of infection.
  - **Inactivated or subunit vaccines**: Safer for immunocompromised patients and generally recommended, although the immune response may be reduced.
- Vaccination protocols :
  - **Initial assessment**: Assess immunisation status, type and degree of immunosuppression, and risk of exposure to infectious agents.
  - **Planning**: Draw up an appropriate vaccination schedule, taking into account the recommendations for immunocompromised patients.
  - **Follow-up**: Check the effectiveness of the vaccination with serological tests if necessary, and consider booster doses.
- Special precautions :
  - **Avoid live vaccines**: With certain exceptions or in special situations.
  - **Post-vaccination monitoring**: Monitor patients closely for adverse reactions or signs of infection.
  - **Communication**: Inform the patient of the benefits and risks, and explain the importance of reporting any unusual symptoms after vaccination.
- Education and awareness :
  - **Information**: Provide clear information on vaccines, their importance, potential side-effects and precautions to be taken.
  - **Patient involvement**: Encourage patients to take an active role in their health, to ask

questions and to adhere to the vaccination schedule.
- **Support**: Offer emotional support, especially when the patient is worried or hesitant about vaccination.

Immunocompromised patients present unique challenges when it comes to vaccination. Their care requires a thorough understanding of immunological principles, effective communication and attention to detail. The nurse, in close collaboration with the attending physician, is an essential pillar in ensuring that these patients receive the appropriate vaccines safely and effectively.

Advice
to avoid allergenic exposure

Allergens, which are omnipresent in our environment, can trigger a variety of reactions in sensitive individuals. It is essential for allergy sufferers to understand how to minimise exposure to these substances to reduce the risk of symptoms and exacerbations. Here is some practical advice, broken down according to different environments and situations, that allergist nurses can pass on to their patients.

- At home :
    - **Dust mites**: Use anti-dust mite covers for mattresses, pillows and duvets. Wash bedding regularly at a high temperature. Maintain low humidity with dehumidifiers if necessary.
    - **Pets**: If you are allergic, avoid adopting furry or feathered animals. If you already have one, keep it out of your bedroom and wash it regularly. Remember to vacuum frequently.

- **Pollens**: Keep windows closed during pollen peaks, use the air conditioning in "recirculation" mode. Rinse your hair in the evening to remove pollen.
- **Mould**: Ensure good ventilation, repair leaks quickly and use dehumidifiers in damp areas.
- Outside :
  - **Pollens**: Avoid outdoor activities during pollen peaks, wear sunglasses to protect your eyes, and check the pollen forecast regularly.
  - **Insect bites**: Wear covering clothing, avoid perfumes and use repellents if you are in a high-risk area.
- At work :
  - **Common allergens** : Tell your employer about your allergies. If possible, adapt your environment (for example, stay away from laser printers if you are allergic to the particles they emit).
  - **Personal protection**: Use masks, gloves or other protective equipment if you are exposed to specific allergens in the course of your work.
- Power supply :
  - **Labelling**: Always read food labels to identify the presence of allergens.
  - **Restaurants**: Always tell the staff about your allergies. Choose places that are used to dealing with food allergies.
- Travel :
  - **Preparation**: Take your allergy medication with you, find out about common allergens at your destination, and consider wearing a medical alert bracelet.
  - **Accommodation**: If possible, choose hotels or accommodation with hypoallergenic rooms.

- Education and awareness :
    - **Learn to recognise**: Familiarise yourself with common allergens and their sources. This will help you avoid them more effectively.
    - **Action plan**: Together with your doctor or nurse, draw up an allergy action plan detailing the steps to be taken in the event of exposure or reaction.

The prevention of allergenic exposure relies as much on modifying the environment as on educating the patient. An informed and proactive patient can greatly reduce the risk of exposure and, as a result, improve quality of life.

Awareness programmes for the general public

Raising public awareness is crucial to preventing allergic diseases, improving their management and reducing the complications associated with them. The more people are informed, the more they can take steps to avoid allergens, recognise the symptoms of an allergic reaction and know how to intervene in an emergency. Here is a detailed presentation of awareness programmes for the general public, their importance and their key components.

- Objectives of awareness programmes :
    - **Educate**: Provide the public with accurate, up-to-date information on allergies, their causes, symptoms and treatments.
    - **Prevent**: Reduce the incidence of new allergies and minimise the complications of existing allergies.
    - **Support**: Offering support to allergy sufferers and their families.

- **Promote** : Encouraging good practice in the management of allergies, whether at home, at school, at work or in other contexts.
- Programme types :
  - **Educational workshops**: Organised in schools, community centres and other public spaces to teach people how to recognise and manage allergies.
  - **Media campaigns**: Use of television, radio, press and social media to disseminate key allergy messages.
  - **Awareness days**: Annual or one-off events, such as World Allergy Day, to highlight certain aspects of allergies.
  - **School programmes**: Integrating allergy education into the school curriculum, teaching children the basics of allergies.
- Key components :
  - **Educational material**: Brochures, videos, posters and websites providing reliable information on allergies.
  - **Training courses**: For teachers, employers and other professionals to help them understand and manage allergies in their context.
  - **Testimonials**: Personal accounts from people living with allergies to humanise the problem and encourage empathy.
  - **Mentoring programmes**: Putting newly-diagnosed people in touch with people who have been living with allergies for a long time to offer support and advice.
- Assessment and improvement :
  - **Monitoring and evaluation**: Collecting data on the effectiveness of programmes to ensure they are achieving their objectives.

- **Updates**: Regularly review programme content to ensure it is up to date with the latest research and recommendations.
- **Feedback**: Gathering comments from the public and participants to continually improve the programmes.

- Collaboration :
  - **Partnerships**: Working with other organisations, healthcare professionals, educators and decision-makers to extend the reach and impact of the programmes.
  - **Networking**: Create and maintain networks with other awareness-raising organisations to share resources, ideas and best practice.

Allergy awareness programmes are essential to inform the general public, prevent complications and support those affected. By combining education, prevention and support, these programmes can play a major role in improving public health and the quality of life of allergy sufferers.

Chapter 7:
THERAPEUTIC PROCEDURES

Allergen immunotherapy

Allergen immunotherapy, often called "desensitisation", is a therapeutic approach aimed at modifying the body's immune response to a specific allergen, gradually reducing its sensitivity. It is one of the few interventions that addresses not only the symptoms of allergies, but also the underlying cause. Here is a detailed exploration of this approach, its mechanisms, indications and application in medical practice.

- **Basic principle :**
  The aim of immunotherapy is to gradually accustom the immune system to a specific allergen, by regularly administering increasing doses of the allergen until a maintenance dose is reached. This leads to a reduction in allergic symptoms on subsequent exposure to the allergen.
- Mechanisms of action :
  - **Modification of the immune response**: Immunotherapy promotes the production of specific immunoglobulin G (IgG), which binds to the allergen before it can trigger an allergic reaction.
  - **Reduced histamine production**: By reducing sensitivity to allergens, the body releases less histamine, a molecule involved in many allergic symptoms.
  - **T-cell regulation**: Immunotherapy modifies the T-cell response, thereby reducing allergic inflammation.

- **Indications** :
  Immunotherapy is mainly recommended for :
    - Pollen allergies.
    - Dust mite allergies.
    - Allergies to insect venoms.
    - Certain forms of allergic asthma.
- It is not generally used for food allergies, except in certain specific cases.
- Methods of administration :
    - **Subcutaneous (SCIT)**: The allergen is injected under the skin, usually into the arm. This is the oldest and most common method.
    - **Sublingual (SLIT)**: The allergen is administered in the form of drops or tablets placed under the tongue. This method is becoming increasingly popular due to the ease with which it can be administered at home.
- **Duration and frequency**:
  Treatment generally begins with an escalation phase, in which the dose is increased regularly. Once the maintenance dose has been reached, it is administered regularly, often for 3 to 5 years.
- **Effectiveness and benefits** :
  Immunotherapy can significantly reduce allergic symptoms, reduce the need for medication and improve quality of life. For some patients, the benefits may persist even after treatment has ended.
- **Side effects**:
  While local reactions such as redness or swelling at the injection site are common, more serious systemic reactions may occur, although these are rare. Monitoring after administration, especially for the first few doses, is essential.
- **Contraindications and precautions**:
  Immunotherapy is not recommended for people suffering from certain heart diseases or immune

disorders, or for pregnant women, unless medical advice indicates otherwise.

Allergen immunotherapy is a powerful and transformative approach for many allergy sufferers. However, careful assessment by an allergist is essential to determine the suitability of the treatment, as well as to ensure its safe administration.

Biological treatments in immunology

Recent advances in biotechnology have paved the way for a new generation of medical treatments: biological treatments. In immunology, these treatments are having a considerable impact, offering promising therapeutic alternatives for diseases that were previously difficult to treat. Biological treatments are distinguished by their origin (often derived from living cells) and their targeted mechanism of action. Let's find out more about this revolution in immunology.

- **Definition of biological treatments**:
  Unlike traditional medicines, which are chemically synthesised, biological treatments are produced from living cells. These drugs specifically target certain parts of the immune system, modulating its response.
- Mechanisms of action :
    - **Monoclonal antibodies**: These molecules mimic the natural antibodies produced by the immune system, but are designed to specifically target certain cells or proteins.
    - **Inhibitors**: These treatments block specific proteins that play a role in inflammation or the immune response.

- **Immune response modifiers**: These agents adjust the activity of the immune system, either stimulating it or reducing it.
- Applications in immunology :
  - **Autoimmune diseases**: such as rheumatoid arthritis, psoriasis or ankylosing spondylitis. Biological treatments can target specific cytokines or immune cells to reduce inflammation and disease progression.
  - **Immunodeficiency**: Certain biological treatments can be used to stimulate or strengthen the immune system.
  - **Allergic diseases**: Biologics can target cytokines or other molecules involved in allergic responses.
- Advantages :
  - **Precision**: Biological treatments are designed to specifically target precise components of the immune system, which can reduce side effects.
  - **Effectiveness**: For many patients, biologics offer relief when other treatments have failed.
  - **New hope**: These treatments open the door to therapies for diseases previously considered untreatable.
- **Precautions and side effects**:
  Although biologics offer many benefits, they can also present risks. Side effects can include infections, injection site reactions and, in rare cases, serious illnesses such as tuberculosis or cancer. Regular monitoring is essential.
- **The future of biological treatments**:
  With ongoing research and the development of new technologies, the future of biological treatments in immunology is promising. New drugs and new applications are constantly being studied, offering the hope of a better quality of life for many patients.

Biological treatments represent a major advance in immunology, transforming the therapeutic landscape and offering new options for patients. As with any medical intervention, a careful assessment of the benefits and risks is essential to ensure the safe and effective use of these powerful tools.

Treatment
the side effects of treatment

When it comes to treating allergic and immunological conditions, the main aim is to relieve patients' symptoms and improve their quality of life. However, as with most medical treatments, there can be side effects. Effective management of these effects is essential to ensure the patient's well-being throughout the course of treatment.

- Recognition and documentation :
  - **Regular monitoring**: Nurses must regularly assess patients to detect any new symptoms or changes in health that could be linked to the treatment.
  - **Symptom diary**: Encouraging patients to keep a detailed diary of their symptoms can help identify side effects and adjust treatment accordingly.
- Patient education :
  - **Information on potential side effects**: Before starting treatment, it is essential to inform the patient of possible side effects and what to expect.
  - **Self-monitoring**: Teaching patients to recognise the signs and symptoms of common side effects and to know when to consult a healthcare professional.

- Symptomatic management :
    - **Complementary treatments**: In some cases, additional drugs may be prescribed to specifically manage side effects, such as antiemetics for nausea.
    - **Non-drug therapies**: Approaches such as physiotherapy, relaxation or dietetics can help manage certain side effects.
- Adjustment of treatment :
    - **Modification of doses**: If side effects are moderate, it may be possible to reduce the dose of the drug while maintaining its efficacy.
    - **Change of treatment** : In situations where side effects are severe or intolerable, it may be necessary to consider other treatment options.
- Psychological support :
    - **Managing anxiety and stress**: Fear of side effects can be a source of anxiety for many patients. Offering a listening ear, support and resources, such as support groups, can be beneficial.
    - **Decision-making support**: Nurses can play an essential role in discussing the advantages and disadvantages of each treatment with patients, helping them to make informed decisions.
- Communication with the care team :
    - **Regular reports**: Nurses must regularly inform the care team of the patient's condition and any side effects observed.
    - **Multidisciplinary collaboration**: Working in close collaboration with other health professionals (doctors, pharmacists, nutritionists) means that side effects can be managed holistically.

Although the side effects of allergology and immunology treatments can sometimes be unavoidable, proper management can greatly improve patient well-being. Nurses play a crucial role in this management, acting as educators, advocates and carers for their patients.

Recent advances in terms of treatment

Allergology and immunology are dynamic medical fields, constantly enriched by new scientific discoveries and technological advances. These advances are revolutionising the way we approach, diagnose and treat allergies and immune disorders. Let's take a look at some of the most significant recent advances in this field.

- **Targeted therapies**:
  Thanks to a better understanding of the underlying molecular mechanisms of allergic and immune diseases, targeted therapies have been developed. These treatments are designed to act on specific pathways involved in the disease, thereby minimising side effects.
    - **Monoclonal antibodies**: Used to specifically target cytokines or other key molecules in the allergic or inflammatory response.
    - **Small molecules**: These compounds can inhibit specific enzyme pathways involved in immune processes.
- **Personalised immunotherapy**:
  Advances in genomics and molecular biology mean that immunotherapy can be tailored to the specific needs of each patient, based on their genetic and immunological profiles.
- **Microbiota and immunology**:
  The discovery of the importance of the intestinal microbiota in regulating the immune system has

opened up new therapeutic avenues, such as the use of probiotics and prebiotics to modulate the immune response.

- **Gene therapy** :
  For patients with inherited immune deficiencies, gene therapy offers the promise of correcting the genetic defect at source. Although this approach is still in its infancy, it has shown promising results in specific cases.

- **Cell therapies**:
  Treatments such as haematopoietic stem cells can be used to rebuild a failing immune system, particularly for patients with severe immune deficiencies.

- **Biotherapies and nanotechnologies**:
  The use of nanoparticles to administer drugs or modulate the immune response is a fast-growing area of research. Nanotechnologies can enable targeted drug delivery, reducing side effects and increasing efficacy.

- **Digital platforms and telemedicine**:
  With the evolution of technology, telemedicine has become a reality for many patients. It allows regular monitoring, remote symptom management and disease education, especially in remote areas.

- **Education and prevention programmes**:
  Recognising the importance of prevention, many new programmes are being set up to educate the public, raise awareness of the importance of allergies and immune disorders and offer advice on how to manage them.

Recent advances in allergy and immunology treatments offer renewed hope to patients and healthcare professionals. As research progresses, it is likely that we will continue to see the emergence of more effective, safer and more personalised treatments.

Chapter 8:
INTERDISCIPLINARY COLLABORATION

Work
with other medical specialities

Allergology and immunology are disciplines which, because of their interconnected nature with other systems in the body, require close collaboration with other medical specialities. Nurses specialising in these fields are often called upon to work in tandem with other health professionals to offer patients holistic care.

- **Pneumology:**
  Allergic respiratory conditions such as asthma require joint management with pulmonologists. Lung tests, treatment protocols and crisis intervention require close collaboration.
- **Dermatology:**
  Skin allergies, such as atopic eczema or urticaria, often involve collaboration with dermatologists, who can offer specialist advice on topical treatment and skin protection.
- **Gastroenterology:**
  Food allergies can manifest as gastrointestinal symptoms. Gastroenterologists can help diagnose and treat these symptoms and advise on appropriate diets.
- **Rheumatology:**
  Autoimmune diseases, such as rheumatoid arthritis or lupus, may require joint management with a rheumatologist, who has specific expertise in treating these conditions.

- **Endocrinology**:
  Certain autoimmune diseases can affect the endocrine glands, such as the thyroid. In these cases, collaboration with an endocrinologist is essential.
- **Paediatrics**:
  Children suffering from allergies or immune deficiencies require specific care adapted to their age. Working with a paediatrician ensures that care is tailored to their development.
- **Otorhinolaryngology**:
  Allergies can often manifest themselves through ENT symptoms, such as allergic rhinitis. Working with otorhinolaryngologists enables us to deal with these symptoms in a comprehensive way.
- **Pharmacy**:
  Pharmacists play a crucial role in medicines management, helping to monitor drug interactions, advising on dosage and educating patients on the correct use of medicines.
- **Psychology/Psychiatry**:
  Living with a chronic illness or severe allergy can have an impact on a patient's mental health. Working with psychologists or psychiatrists can help address these issues.
- Dietetics :

For patients with food allergies, a dietician can provide valuable advice on how to maintain a balanced diet while avoiding allergens.

In summary, in the complex world of allergology and immunology, multidisciplinary collaboration is not only beneficial, but often essential. Nurses, as the cornerstone of care teams, play a central role in coordinating this collaboration, ensuring that patients receive comprehensive and integrated care.

The importance of care coordination

Care coordination is an essential aspect of modern medicine, particularly in areas such as allergology and immunology where patients may present with a range of symptoms that straddle several medical specialities. It aims to ensure comprehensive, efficient and patient-centred care, avoiding duplication, medical errors and gaps in care.

- **Optimising resources**:
  Coordination allows available resources to be used optimally. This avoids duplication of examinations, reduces costs for healthcare systems and patients, and ensures that resources are used where they are most needed.
- **Continuity of care**:
  Continuous care is crucial for patients with chronic conditions. Thanks to effective coordination, patient information flows seamlessly between the various healthcare professionals, ensuring uninterrupted care.
- **Patient safety**:
  Coordination reduces the risk of medical errors, undetected drug interactions and contraindications. Patients benefit from consistent treatment based on complete, up-to-date information.
- **Holistic care**:
  By understanding a patient's whole clinical picture, carers can address not only the physical symptoms, but also the patient's emotional, social and psychological needs.
- **Patient education and empowerment**:
  Good care coordination also involves educating patients about their condition, the treatment options available and the day-to-day management of their

health. This makes them more independent and able to actively participate in their own care.

- **Time efficiency**:
  Care coordination enables smooth communication between healthcare professionals. This reduces the time spent searching for information, clarifying uncertainties and organising appointments, making care more efficient.
- **Patient satisfaction**:
  Patients who feel that their care is smoothly coordinated are generally more satisfied with their care. They feel they are listened to, respected and cared for as a whole.
- **Updating treatment protocols**:
  Care coordination also ensures that treatment protocols are regularly updated in line with the latest medical advances. This ensures that patients benefit from the latest and most effective treatments.
- **Reducing Care Fragmentation**:
  Without coordination, care can become fragmented, with different specialists prescribing treatments without knowledge of other ongoing interventions. Coordination ensures a unified approach.
- Optimising Medical Outcomes :

Ultimately, effective care coordination means better medical outcomes for patients. Treatments are more consistent, complications are minimised, and patients benefit from comprehensive, holistic care.

Care coordination is therefore an essential link in the medical care chain. For allergy and immunology nurses, this is particularly important given the complexity of the conditions treated and the need for multidisciplinary care.

Communicating effectively with doctors, pharmacists and other healthcare professionals

Communication is an essential skill for any healthcare professional. In the dynamic and interdisciplinary context of allergology and immunology, nurses must work closely with a variety of specialists to ensure optimal patient care. Effective communication ensures safety, patient satisfaction and effective care. Here are some tips and techniques for successful communication:

- Active listening :
    - Be present during the exchange, concentrate on the speaker.
    - Don't formulate answers before the other person has finished.
    - Ask questions to clarify ambiguous points.
- Clarify medical terms:
    - Use simple language when talking to professionals from other specialities to avoid any confusion.
    - Ask for clarification if a term or instruction is unclear.
- Use structured communication tools:
    - Methods such as SBAR (Situation, Background, Assessment, Recommendation) can help to structure communication, particularly in urgent situations.
- Be respectful and open:
    - Recognising the expertise and perspective of other team members.
    - Avoid hasty judgements or unconstructive criticism.

- Precise documentation :
  - Ensure that all relevant information is clearly and concisely documented in the patient's medical record.
  - Written notes are often used as a means of communication between healthcare professionals.
- Interdisciplinary team meeting :
  - Actively participate in team meetings to discuss patients, share information and develop care plans.
  - These meetings provide an opportunity to discuss complex cases in depth.
- Use technology to your advantage:
  - Electronic communication platforms, electronic medical records and telemedicine tools can facilitate rapid communication between professionals.
- Give and receive feedback:
  - Feedback is essential for continuous improvement. If a communication strategy is proving ineffective, look for ways to improve it.
- Develop a basic knowledge of other specialities:
  - By understanding the roles and responsibilities of other members of the care team, you can better anticipate their needs and questions.
- Build solid relationships:
- The time invested in building solid and respectful professional relationships with other members of the medical team will result in more fluid and effective communication.

Effective communication is at the heart of interdisciplinary care. Nurses, as central members of the care team, must master this skill to ensure patient safety, consistent care and optimal outcomes. By adopting sound communication techniques and building relationships based on mutual respect, nurses can make a significant contribution to excellence in care.

Chapter 9:
SPECIFIC INSTRUMENTS AND EQUIPMENT

Introduction to specific tools in Allergology and Immunology

Allergology and immunology, being constantly evolving medical fields, use a range of specific tools to diagnose, treat and monitor patients. These tools, whether technological or practical, are essential for providing accurate and personalised care. This introduction provides an overview of the instruments and techniques commonly used by professionals in these disciplines.

- **Skin tests**:
  These tests involve applying small amounts of potential allergens to the skin, usually on the forearm or back, to assess the allergic reaction.
    - **Prick test**: A drop of the allergen is placed on the skin, which is then pricked lightly with a needle.
    - **Patch test**: The allergen is applied under an occlusive dressing for 48 hours, ideal for contact allergens.
- **Spirometry**:
  An essential tool for assessing lung function. Patients blow into a spirometer, which measures the volume and speed of air inhaled and exhaled. It is frequently used to diagnose and monitor asthma.
- **Immunoglobulin E (IgE) test**:
  A blood test used to measure the level of IgE specific to a particular allergen, aiding in the diagnosis of allergies.

- **Provocation tests**:
  Under close supervision, the patient is exposed to a suspected allergen under controlled conditions to observe any reaction.
- **Immunotherapy**:
  A treatment that gradually exposes the patient to increasing doses of a specific allergen to reduce sensitivity.
- Biological tests :
  - **Flow cytometry**: A technique for analysing and sorting cells, essential for studying sub-populations of immune cells.
  - **Neutrophil function test**: Assesses the ability of neutrophils to engulf and kill bacteria.
- **Lymphoblastic Transformation Test** :
  Assesses the response of lymphocytes to different stimuli, often used to diagnose certain immunodeficiencies.
- **Medical imaging**:
  Techniques such as chest X-rays or CT scans can be used to assess complications related to allergies or autoimmune diseases.
- **Electronic Medical Records (EMR)**:
  A digital tool for recording, storing and sharing patient medical information. The EMR facilitates the coordination of care between different healthcare professionals.
- **Applications and Monitoring Tools** :
  Numerous applications allow patients to record their symptoms and allergic triggers, or to monitor their lung function at home.
- **New biological treatments** :
  These are drugs derived from biological sources, specifically designed to target certain parts of the immune system. They are increasingly used in the treatment of autoimmune diseases and certain severe allergies.

- **Educational tools :**

Brochures, videos and workshops for patients and their families to inform them about their condition, the treatments available and self-management strategies.

These tools, combined with the clinical expertise of healthcare professionals, enable a comprehensive and personalised approach to allergology and immunology care. Mastery of these tools is therefore crucial for any nurse working in these specialities.

Maintenance, sterilisation, and safe use

The integrity, sterilisation and safety of the tools and equipment used in allergology and immunology are crucial to ensuring high-quality medical care and minimising the risk of infection. Poor maintenance or ineffective sterilisation can lead to serious complications for patients.

- Basic principles :
    - **Hand hygiene**: This is the first line of defence against infection. Washing your hands before and after handling any equipment is essential.
    - **Wearing personal protective equipment**: Gloves, masks, gowns and safety glasses may be necessary depending on the situation.
- Regular equipment   maintenance :
    - Ensure that all equipment is regularly inspected and maintained in accordance with the manufacturer's recommendations.
    - Any faulty equipment must be immediately removed from the care chain.
- Sterilisation :
    - Reusable instruments must be cleaned and sterilised after each use. Autoclaves, which use

pressurised steam to kill micro-organisms, are commonly used for this task.

- Disinfection solutions can be used for certain equipment, but they must be changed regularly and used in accordance with the manufacturer's instructions.

- Use of single-use instruments :
  - Many allergology and immunology instruments are single-use to avoid the risk of cross-infection.
  - These instruments must be disposed of properly after use in appropriate containers.

- Training and awareness :
  - Nursing and medical staff must be regularly trained and made aware of sterilisation and maintenance protocols.
  - Periodic audits and evaluations can help to identify shortcomings or areas for improvement.

- Secure storage :
  - Sterilised instruments must be stored in a clean, dry environment, free from contamination.
  - Cabinets and storage areas must be regularly cleaned and disinfected.

- Traceability :
  - Keeping detailed records of equipment, maintenance and use can help ensure traceability and identify any irregularities quickly.

- Waste management :
  - Biomedical waste, such as needles and other sharp instruments, must be disposed of safely in appropriate containers.
  - Waste must be disposed of in accordance with local regulations.

- Patient and staff safety :
  - Make sure all equipment is working properly and safely to minimise risks to patients and staff.
- Continuous assessment :
  - Medical technology is evolving rapidly. It is therefore essential to continually evaluate the tools and techniques used to ensure that they remain at the cutting edge of technology and in line with best practice.

Rigorous management of allergology and immunology equipment is essential to ensure the safety of patients and staff. The maintenance, sterilisation and safe use of tools are fundamental aspects of the quality of care and infection prevention.

Technological innovations and their impact on practice

In this age of technology and personalised medicine, allergology and immunology are benefiting from revolutionary advances that are transforming patient care. These innovations are not only improving the quality of care, but also making life easier for healthcare professionals and patients.

- **Teleconsultation** :
  With the rise of telemedicine, remote consultations have become possible. This gives patients access to specialists without having to travel, especially those living in remote areas.
- **Mobile applications**:
  Patients can use apps to monitor their symptoms, take medication on time or even perform lung function tests at home. This data can then be shared

with healthcare professionals for more personalised monitoring.

- **Wearable Technologies**:
Wearable devices such as watches and bracelets can now monitor vital parameters such as heart rate or oxygen saturation, alerting patients and doctors to any abnormalities.
- **Artificial Intelligence (AI)**:
AI can help analyse test results, predict allergic reactions or detect autoimmune diseases at an early stage. It offers assistance in diagnosis and therapeutic decision-making.
- **Gene therapy**:
Although still in the research phase for certain diseases, gene therapy could offer curative treatments for certain immune diseases by modifying the genetic code.
- **3D printing**:
This enables the creation of three-dimensional models of organs or immune systems, facilitating patient education and medical training.
- **Biotechnology**:
Advances in this field have led to the creation of biological drugs that specifically target certain parts of the immune system, offering more effective treatments with fewer side effects.
- **Electronic Medical   Records (EMR)**:
A more advanced version of EMRs, incorporating AI, could help with early detection of complications, analysis of patient data and better coordination of care.
- **Online educational platforms**:
Nurses, doctors and patients can access resources, training and webinars to keep abreast of the latest developments.

- Virtual reality   tools :

Used for medical training or to help patients understand their illness, these immersive tools offer a unique learning experience.

The impact of these innovations on medical practice is immense. They enable earlier diagnosis, more personalised care and improve patients' quality of life. However, it is essential that healthcare professionals receive adequate training to use these technologies effectively. In addition, ethical and regulatory considerations must be taken into account, particularly with regard to the protection of patient data.

Training and skills required to use the instruments

Mastery of the instruments and equipment specific to allergology and immunology is essential to guarantee patient safety and accurate diagnosis and treatment. This requires appropriate training and the development of specific skills.

- Academic and clinical training :
    - **Nursing degree**: The starting point is usually a nursing degree, which provides an introduction to the basic skills needed to work in a medical environment.
    - **Specialist   training**: Additional training in allergology and immunology is often recommended for those wishing to specialise in this field.
- Workshops and practical training :
    - **Clinical placements**: Nurses must complete placements in specialised clinics or hospitals to gain practical experience.

- **Workshops and seminars**: Equipment manufacturers and professional associations often organise workshops to train nurses in the use of new instruments or technologies.
- Technical skills :
  - **Equipment handling**: Knowing how to use, maintain and troubleshoot equipment specific to allergology and immunology.
  - **Test procedures**: mastering skin test procedures, spirometry, vaccine administration and other routine procedures.
- Safety skills :
  - **Sterilisation protocols**: Knowledge of the appropriate sterilisation methods for each instrument.
  - **Infection prevention**: Understanding and following protocols to prevent cross-infection.
- Continuous updating :
  - **Ongoing training**: With the rapid development of medical technologies, it is essential to take regular training courses to keep abreast of the latest advances.
- Communication skills :
  - **Interpreting results**: Ability to read, understand and communicate test results to doctors and patients.
  - **Patient education**: Explaining procedures, treatments and outcomes to patients in a clear and empathetic manner.
- Management skills :
  - **Organisation**: managing time effectively, organising appointments and coordinating with other healthcare professionals.
  - **Accurate documentation**: Keeping medical records up to date, documenting test results and interventions.

- Professional development :
  - **Certifications and specialisations**: Obtaining certifications in specific fields, such as allergen immunotherapy, can enhance skills and credibility.
- Critical thinking and decision-making :
  - Analysing situations, interpreting data and making informed decisions for the patient's well-being.
- Adaptability :
- With technology and medical protocols constantly evolving, it's essential to be flexible and ready to learn and adapt.

The safe and effective use of instruments in allergology and immunology requires a combination of formal training, practical training, technical skills and interpersonal skills. Continuous development of these skills ensures that patients receive the best possible care.

Chapter 10:
MANAGING COMPLEX SITUATIONS

Refractory patients
to standard treatments

In the field of allergology and immunology, some patients may not respond to standard or commonly used treatments, thus qualifying as "refractory patients". Understanding and managing these patients is a major challenge for healthcare professionals.

- **What is a refractory patient?**
  A refractory patient is one who does not respond to initial treatment or who relapses after an initial response. This non-response may be due to a variety of factors, including the severity of the disease, the presence of multiple co-morbidities, or genetic variations.
- Causes of refractoriness:
    - **Individual characteristics**: Each patient is unique, and their genetics, metabolism or environment may affect their response to treatment.
    - **Non-compliance with treatment**: Poor adherence to treatment, often due to side effects, can be a cause.
    - **Complexity   of the disease**: Allergies and autoimmune diseases can present in complex forms, making some cases more difficult to treat.
- **Identification of refractory patients**:
  Regular monitoring of symptoms, use of diagnostic

90

tests, and assessment of response to treatment are essential to identify these patients.

- Therapeutic approaches for refractory patients:
    - **Modification of treatment**: Increase in dose, change of medication, or combination of several treatments.
    - **Biological treatments**: Certain biological drugs can specifically target parts of the immune system involved in the disease.
    - **Immunotherapy**: For some allergy sufferers, immunotherapy can help to desensitise the immune system.
    - **Non-pharmacological interventions**: Psychotherapy, rehabilitation or stress management techniques can complement medical treatment.
- Challenges associated with management:
    - **Side-effects**: Alternative or intensified treatments may have more marked side-effects.
    - **Cost**: Some treatments for refractory patients can be expensive, posing challenges in terms of reimbursement or access.
    - **Emotional burden**: Refractoriness can be stressful and depressing for patients, requiring psychological support.
- **Interdisciplinary collaboration**:
The management of refractory patients may require close collaboration between allergists, immunologists, psychologists, and other specialists for a holistic approach.
- **Research and clinical trials**:
Refractory patients may have the opportunity to take part in clinical trials for new treatments. This is also an incentive for ongoing research in the field.
- **Patient education and support**:
It is essential to involve the patient in the decision-

making process, to inform them of the options available, and to support them emotionally.

Refractory patients in allergology and immunology represent a major clinical challenge, but also an opportunity to deepen our understanding of these diseases and to innovate in terms of treatment. Personalised management, inter-professional collaboration and ongoing research are essential to provide the best possible care for these patients.

Allergies and immunodepressions in paediatric patients

Children are not simply little adults; their immune systems develop and evolve over time. As a result, the management of allergies and immunodepressions in paediatric patients often differs from that of adults. Let's approach this subject with precision, sensitivity and a concern for medical integrity.

- Understanding the basics:
    - **Development of the immune system**: From birth, and as they grow, children are exposed to a multitude of antigens that shape their immune system.
    - **Genetic and environmental factors**: genes inherited from parents and the environment play a decisive role in the development of allergies and immune deficiencies.
- Paediatric allergies:
    - **Food allergies**: Includes diagnosis, management and prevention of common allergies such as those to milk, eggs, peanuts, etc.

- **Atopic eczema**: A common condition in infants and children.
- **Asthma**: The symptoms and management of asthma in children often differ from those in adults.
- **Seasonal allergies**: Reactions to pollen, moulds and other allergens in the environment.
- Paediatric immunodepression:
    - **Primary immune deficiencies**: These deficiencies are generally genetic and can affect different components of the immune system.
    - **Secondary immune deficiencies**: These can occur as a result of infections, drug treatments or other medical conditions.
    - **Opportunistic infections**: In immunocompromised children, infections that are generally benign can become serious.
- Diagnose and assess:
    - **Clinical presentation**: Symptoms of allergies and immune deficiencies in children.
    - **Diagnostic tests**: Skin tests, blood tests and other procedures suitable for children.
- Specific treatments for children:
    - **Medicines**: Dosages, methods of administration and side effects in children.
    - **Therapeutic education**: How to teach children and their families the best ways to manage their conditions.
    - **Adherence to treatment**: Ensuring the follow-up and cooperation of young patients.
- Prevention and education:
    - **Vaccinations**: The essential role of vaccines, especially in immunocompromised children.
    - **Avoiding allergens**: Tips for parents on avoiding exposure to common allergens.

- **Nutrition and diet**: The importance of a healthy diet and specific diets for allergic children.
- Psychosocial challenges and support:
    - **Impact on the family**: Caring for a child with allergies or immunodepression can be stressful for the whole family.
    - **Psychological support**: The importance of emotional support for children and their families.
    - **School and social activities**: How to help an allergic or immunocompromised child to live normally at school and in other social environments.

The management of allergies and immunodepressions in children requires a comprehensive and integrated approach, adapted to the specific needs of paediatrics. Working closely with children, their families, schools and other stakeholders is essential to ensure their well-being, safety and quality of life.

Care for elderly patients

With advancing age, the immune system undergoes structural and functional changes, known as immunosenescence. Elderly patients can present unique challenges in allergology and immunology, requiring an approach tailored to their specific needs.

- Immunosenescence and its implications:
    - **Changes in the immune system with age**: Understanding how the immune system changes with age, and how this impacts susceptibility to disease and infection.

- **Increased vulnerability**: Elderly patients are often more vulnerable to infections and may experience atypical allergic reactions.
- Allergies in elderly patients:
  - **Clinical manifestations**: Allergic symptoms may be attenuated, atypical or masked by other conditions common in the elderly.
  - **Triggers**: Exploration of common allergens and how they affect the elderly.
- Immunosuppression in elderly patients:
  - **Causes and consequences**: Immune deficiencies can be amplified by other chronic diseases, drug treatments and immunosenescence.
  - **Management**: The importance of appropriate assessment and monitoring to minimise risks.
- Diagnosis in elderly patients:
  - **Special challenges**: Standard tests may need to be adjusted or interpreted differently.
  - **Importance of the history**: A careful history is essential, given the likelihood of co-morbidities and concomitant medications.
- Treatments adapted to elderly patients:
  - **Medicines and dosages**: Take into account changes in pharmacokinetics and pharmacodynamics with age.
  - **Managing side effects**: The elderly may be more sensitive to certain side effects or drug interactions.
- Holistic approach:
  - **Taking co-morbidities into account**: Elderly patients often have a number of concomitant conditions that can influence their management.
  - **Psychosocial aspects**: the importance of emotional support, lifestyle habits and social context.

- Education and prevention:
  - **Adherence to treatment** : Ensuring patient understanding and co-operation, taking into account any cognitive or physical limitations.
  - **Vaccinations**: Vaccination recommendations may differ and are essential to protect the elderly from infections.
- Multidisciplinary collaboration:
  - **Care coordination**: Working with other specialists, such as geriatricians, to provide comprehensive care.
  - **Family and carers**: The essential role of relatives in care, support and decision-making.

The management of elderly patients in allergology and immunology requires an in-depth understanding of age-related changes and the specific challenges associated with this population. A personalised, multidisciplinary and caring approach will ensure optimal care and a better quality of life for these patients.

Challenges linked to rare and orphan diseases

The term 'rare diseases' refers to a broad category of diseases that affect a small percentage of the population. In the context of allergology and immunology, some of these diseases are termed 'orphan' because they do not attract the attention of researchers or the pharmaceutical industry due to their low prevalence. These diseases pose unique challenges for healthcare professionals and patients alike.

- Understanding rare diseases:
    - **Definition and classification**: what is meant by "rare diseases" and how they are classified in allergology and immunology.
    - **Epidemiology**: The prevalence, distribution and evolution of these diseases.
- Diagnosis: A path strewn with pitfalls :
    - **Delays in diagnosis**: Many patients with rare diseases go years without a precise diagnosis.
    - **Complexity of symptoms**: Manifestations may be vague, atypical or resemble other more common conditions.
- Lack of research and data :
    - **Limited funding**: Research into rare diseases is often under-funded because it does not attract commercial interest.
    - **Clinical trials**: Difficulties in conducting robust studies due to the small number of patients.
- Therapeutic challenges :
    - **Limited or non-existent treatments**: Many rare diseases have no specific treatment.
    - **Orphan drugs**: The challenges and hopes involved in developing drugs for these diseases.
- Comprehensive patient care :
    - **Multidisciplinary approach**: The need for close collaboration between various specialists to address all aspects of the disease.
    - **Psychological support**: Recognising and dealing with the emotional and psychological impact on patients and their families.
- Education and awareness :
    - **Training healthcare professionals**: Ensuring that carers are well informed and prepared to identify and manage these diseases.

- **Raising public awareness**: Increasing the visibility of these diseases to attract attention, funding and research.
- Collaboration and networks :
  - **Reference centres**: The importance of specialised centres to provide expert care.
  - **Patient networks** : Patient associations play a crucial role in providing support, information and campaigning for research.
- Ethical and social aspects :
  - **Access to care**: Ensuring that all patients, regardless of their geographical or socio-economic situation, have access to treatment and care.
  - **Ethical issues**: prenatal diagnosis, genetics and the end of life.

Rare and orphan diseases in allergology and immunology require special attention. Although they affect a small percentage of the population, the impact on affected individuals and their families is profound. A holistic, patient-centred approach, combined with vigorous research, is essential to improve diagnosis, treatment and quality of life for these patients.

Chapter 11:
ALLERGOLOGY RESEARCH
AND IMMUNOLOGY

The importance of clinical research and fundamental

Allergology and immunology, like all medical disciplines, are based on decades, even centuries, of research. Innovation, exploration and understanding continue to evolve through the combined efforts of basic and clinical research. These two pillars, though distinct in their approaches, are intrinsically linked and are essential to achieving significant improvements in patient care.

- Fundamental research: Exploring the basics :
    - **Definition and scope**: Understanding what basic research is and how it differs from applied research.
    - **Immunological mechanisms**: Study how the immune system functions at a molecular, cellular and systemic level.
    - **Origins of diseases**: Identifying the genetic, environmental and physiological triggers of allergic and immunological diseases.
- Clinical research: From the laboratory to the patient's bedside :
    - **Clinical trial phases**: Understanding the steps involved in testing new therapies, from safety to efficacy.
    - **Epidemiological studies**: Analysing trends, causes and effects of diseases at population level.

- **Research into the effectiveness of treatments**: Evaluating how treatments work in real-life conditions.
- The interface between basic and clinical research :
  - **Knowledge transfer**: How can laboratory discoveries be translated into potential therapies?
  - **Interdisciplinary collaboration**: The importance of combining diverse expertise for innovative, integrative research.
- Impact on treatment and prevention :
  - **New drugs and therapies**: How research is leading to the development of new, more effective and less invasive treatments.
  - **Prevention strategies**: Using research to anticipate and prevent diseases before they occur.
- Research challenges and ethics :
  - **Ethical issues**: considerations surrounding clinical trials, genomics and synthetic biology.
  - **Funding and support**: The challenges associated with obtaining sufficient and sustainable funding for research.
- The future of allergy and immunology research:
  - **Personalised therapies**: Using genetics and precision medicine to tailor treatments to individual needs.
  - **Emerging technologies**: Innovations, such as genome editing and artificial intelligence, that are shaping future research.

Research, both fundamental and clinical, is the driving force behind progress in allergology and immunology. It enables us to constantly improve our understanding of diseases, develop new treatments and push back the frontiers of what medicine can achieve. For healthcare professionals, keeping abreast of the latest advances is essential if they are to offer the best possible care to their patients.

How the nurse can contribute for research

Nurses occupy a unique position in the healthcare field, being both at the heart of clinical care and at the interface between the patient and the medical team. This privileged position enables them to play a crucial role in research, particularly in Allergology and Immunology.

- Data collection role :
    - **In-depth clinical note-taking**: By carefully documenting patients' symptoms, reactions to treatment and other relevant observations, nurses provide essential data for clinical research.
    - **Post-treatment follow-up**: Observations on the durability of treatments, the appearance of side-effects or patients' quality of life.
- Liaison between patients and researchers :
    - **Recruiting for clinical trials**: The nurse can identify patients likely to benefit from clinical trials and refer them to these opportunities.
    - **Education and consent**: explaining the purpose, benefits and risks of clinical trials to patients, while obtaining their informed consent.
- Conducting nursing research projects :
    - **Identifying problems**: Based on their clinical experience, nurses can identify areas requiring research or improvement.
    - **Developing and implementing protocols**: Designing small studies to test, for example,

new care procedures or educational interventions.
- Participation in multidisciplinary studies:
  - **Research team**: Working with doctors, researchers, pharmacists and other health professionals.
  - **Contribution of a clinical perspective**: Sharing insights based on day-to-day care experience to improve study design and implementation.
- Publication and distribution:
  - **Writing articles**: sharing the results of research or literature reviews in specialist journals.
  - **Conferences and workshops**: Present findings to peers, take part in debates and keep abreast of the latest advances.
- Continuing education and specialisation :
  - **Courses and qualifications**: Specific training in nursing research.
  - **Advanced degrees**: Pursue postgraduate studies to specialise further in research, such as a master's or doctorate in nursing.
- Evidence-based   research lawyer :
  - **Promoting best practice**: Ensuring that the care provided is based on the most recent and solid evidence.
  - **Feedback on existing protocols**: Suggest improvements based on recent research and feedback.

The role of the nurse in research is therefore diverse and essential. Whether by collecting data, conducting projects or disseminating knowledge, nurses are key players in the advancement of research in Allergology and Immunology. Their contribution ensures that the research is relevant, patient-centred and, above all, applicable to everyday clinical practice.

The latest major discoveries and their involvement

Allergology and immunology are constantly evolving fields. Research is flourishing, regularly leading to discoveries that are transforming the understanding and management of allergic and immune diseases. Here are some of the most significant advances in recent years and their implications for clinical practice:

- **Microbiome and immune health** :
  Discovery: The intestine is home to trillions of microbes (bacteria, viruses, fungi) which play a crucial role in regulating our immune system.
  Implication: These discoveries call into question the way in which allergies and certain autoimmune diseases develop, opening the way to treatments based on modulation of the microbiome, such as probiotics or faecal transplants.
- **Biological therapies for autoimmune and allergic diseases**:
  Discovery: Targeted drugs designed to block specific molecules involved in inflammation and the immune response.
  Implication: These drugs offer more effective and less toxic treatments for diseases such as severe asthma, atopic dermatitis and rheumatoid arthritis.
- **Treatment of anaphylaxis** :
  Discovery: New, more user-friendly adrenaline auto-injectors and training in their use.
  Implication: More rapid and effective administration of adrenaline in the event of anaphylaxis, increasing the chances of survival and reducing complications.
- **Desensitisation to food allergens** :
  Discovery: Oral immunotherapy protocols to gradually desensitise patients allergic to certain foods.
  Implication: People with severe food allergies can

potentially be treated to increase their tolerance to the allergen, thereby reducing the risk of serious reactions.

- **Genetics of immune diseases** :
  Discovery: Identification of specific genes associated with immune diseases, such as primary immune deficiency.
  Implications: Earlier and more accurate diagnosis, and the possibility of gene therapies to treat some of these conditions in the future.
- **Immunotherapy in oncology** :
  Discovery: Using the immune system to attack and eliminate cancer cells.
  Implication: This advance has revolutionised the treatment of certain types of cancer, offering therapeutic options where there was little or no hope.

The impact of these discoveries is vast, offering new treatment perspectives, improving patients' quality of life and, in some cases, providing a cure. It is a reminder of the power of research and its importance in the medical field, as well as the essential role of healthcare professionals, including nurses, in translating these discoveries into beneficial care for patients.

The future of research and emerging fields

Allergology and Immunology, as interconnected fields of medicine, continue to evolve rapidly, and new areas of research are constantly emerging. These areas promise to bring new understanding and potential therapeutic advances. Here's a glimpse of what the future might hold for Allergy and Immunology research:

- Personalised immunotherapy :
    - *Focus*: Tailoring immunotherapeutic treatments to a patient's individual genetic and immunological characteristics.
    - *Potential*: Offer more effective treatments with fewer side effects, leading to a better quality of life.
- Neuroimmunology :
    - *Area of interest*: Study of interactions between the nervous system and the immune system.
    - *Potential*: Understanding the links between stress, depression and immune dysfunction, opening up new avenues for therapeutic approaches.
- Epigenetics of immune diseases :
    - *Focus*: Understanding how environmental factors modify the expression of genes linked to the immune response without changing the DNA itself.
    - *Potential*: Identify new disease mechanisms and new therapeutic targets.
- Microbiome and allergology:
    - *Area of interest*: Studying how changes in the microbiome can influence the prevalence and severity of allergies.
    - *Potential*: Developing interventions to restore or modulate the microbiome in order to prevent or treat allergies.
- CRISPR technologies and gene editing :
    - *Area of interest*: Use of gene-editing techniques to correct or modify the genes responsible for immune disorders.
    - *Potential*: Treating genetic diseases at their root, potentially offering cures for currently incurable conditions.

- Nanotechnology in immunology :
  - *Area of interest*: Use of nanoparticles to administer drugs, vaccines or immune system modulating agents.
  - *Potential*: Increase the effectiveness of treatments while reducing side effects.
- Environmental immunology :
  - *Focus*: Understanding the impact of pollutants, toxins and climate change on the immune system.
  - *Potential*: Prevent and treat diseases associated with environmental factors.

These and other emerging areas define the frontier of research in Allergology and Immunology. Continued investment in these areas can lead to transformational discoveries, improving patient care worldwide. For healthcare professionals, including nurses, keeping abreast of these advances is essential to providing optimal care and guiding patients through the complex landscape of therapeutic options.

Chapter 12:
TRANSITION TO OTHER SPECIALITIES OR ADVANCED POSITIONS

The nurse practitioner in Allergology and Immunology

Nurse practitioners (NPs) play a crucial role in the care of patients with allergic and immunological disorders. Their advanced training, combined with their clinical assessment and therapeutic management skills, make NPs an essential link in the continuum of care offered to these patients.

- Definition and professional recognition :
  - *Origins and evolution of the role of the PI*: A brief history of the development of this profession.
  - *Regulatory framework*: The eligibility, training and certification criteria required to work as a PI.
  - Distinction between nurse and nurse practitioner: clarification of skills and responsibilities.
- Skills and training :
  - *Academic training*: The university course and clinical placements required to become a PI in Allergology and Immunology.
  - *Ongoing training*: The importance of regularly updating knowledge and skills.
- Areas of expertise :
  - *Advanced clinical assessment*: The ability to carry out in-depth examinations and interpret complex results.

- *Prescription therapy*: The ability to initiate, adjust or stop treatments in collaboration with doctors.
- *Monitoring and coordinating care*: Ensuring continuity of care for patients, in collaboration with other health professionals.
- Specific role in Allergology and Immunology :
  - *Care for allergy sufferers*: assessment, diagnosis and follow-up of patients with various allergies.
  - *Immunodeficiency management*: Screening, monitoring and referral of patients with immune deficiencies.
  - *Therapeutic education*: raising awareness of allergens, administering treatments and preventing attacks.
- Challenges and opportunities :
  - *Interprofessional collaboration*: The importance of working in synergy with doctors, pharmacists and other healthcare professionals.
  - *Challenges facing the profession*: regulatory limits, obstacles to professional recognition, and clinical challenges.
  - *Opportunities for the future*: Extending the scope of practice, participating in clinical research and contributing to continuing medical education.
- Clinical cases and testimonials :
  - Real-life stories illustrating the role of PI in Allergology and Immunology, highlighting its impact on improving patient care.

The nurse practitioner in Allergology and Immunology is a pillar of patient care. Their in-depth training and advanced clinical skills enable them to provide high-quality care, fill gaps in healthcare systems and actively contribute to the development of medical practices in this specialist field.

The transition to teaching or training

The career of an Allergy and Immunology nurse is not limited to direct patient care. With experience, many nurses are drawn to the world of teaching, seeking to train the next generation of healthcare professionals in this exciting specialty. This transition, although natural, requires specific preparation and reflection.

- Motivations for teaching :
    - *Giving back* : Contribute to the training and mentoring of future nurses.
    - *Professional satisfaction*: The pleasure of seeing students develop and succeed.
    - *Intellectual stimulation*: Keeping up to date with the latest research and advances in the field.
- Skills and qualities required:
    - *Clinical excellence*: Solid experience and in-depth knowledge of the specialty.
    - *Teaching skills*: Knowing how to pass on knowledge effectively.
    - *Patience and empathy*: Understanding students' individual needs and adapting to their learning pace.
- The different educational pathways :
    - *Academic teaching*: Teaching in nursing training institutions or universities.
    - *Clinical training*: Supervising and mentoring students during their field placements.
    - *Workshops and seminars*: Organising or taking part in ongoing training courses for practising professionals.
- Preparing for the transition :
    - *Teacher training*: Acquiring the necessary teaching skills.

- *Get a mentor*: Benefit from the experience and advice of an experienced teacher.
- *Familiarise yourself with the academic world*: Understand how educational institutions work and what they expect.
- The challenges and rewards of teaching :
  - *Managing student diversity*: Every student is unique, with their own strengths, weaknesses and learning style.
  - *Balance between teaching and clinical practice*: Finding the right balance between remaining active in clinical practice and devoting yourself to teaching.
  - *The joys of teaching*: The rewarding moments when students succeed and demonstrate competence.
- Future prospects :
  - *Progression in the academic hierarchy*: Becoming head of department or programme.
  - *Contribution to nursing education research*: Participate in studies and publications related to nursing education.
  - *Ongoing professional development*: Always seeking to improve teaching methods and techniques.

The transition from nurse to teacher is a rewarding path that offers many opportunities for professional growth. By training and guiding the next generation, these nurse educators play an essential role in the evolution and continuous improvement of the nursing profession.

The nurse researcher or consultant

With the constant evolution of medical knowledge, the need to integrate research into nursing practice has never been more crucial. In addition, with the increasing complexity of healthcare, there is a growing demand for specialist consultants to guide practice and policy. Nurses with expertise in allergy and immunology can therefore diversify as researchers or consultants.

- The nurse researcher :
    - *Role definition*: Dedicated to the design, implementation and analysis of clinical or fundamental studies.
    - *Importance of nursing research*: Contributing to the knowledge base to improve clinical practice and patient outcomes.
    - *Research opportunities*: Studies on the effectiveness of interventions, quality of care, patient education, etc.
    - *Interdisciplinary collaboration*: working with doctors, pharmacists, biologists and other professionals.
    - *Disseminating results*: publishing in specialist journals, presenting at conferences, incorporating findings into continuing education.
- The nurse consultant :
    - *Role definition*: Advanced clinical expertise to guide practices, develop protocols or advise on complex clinical situations.
    - *Areas of consultancy*: Case management, care policies, development of patient education programmes.
    - *Collaboration with other institutions*: hospitals, clinics, educational institutions, pharmaceutical companies.
    - *Ongoing training*: constantly updating its knowledge to offer advice based on the latest evidence.

- Training and skills required :
  - *Specialised training* : Advanced degrees in research, epidemiology, biostatistics or other relevant fields.
  - *Analytical skills*: Ability to design studies, analyse data and evaluate scientific literature.
  - *Effective communication*: Ability to present information clearly, write articles and collaborate with other professionals.
- Challenges and awards :
  - *The need for critical thinking*: constantly questioning established practices and seeking improvements.
  - *Balancing several roles*: Navigating between research, consultation, clinical work and sometimes teaching.
  - *Lasting impact*: The satisfaction of contributing to the improvement of care, the development of the profession and a better quality of life for patients.
- Future prospects :
  - *Leadership opportunities*: Taking on leadership roles in research institutions, professional associations or healthcare organisations.
  - *Expanding the scope of consultation*: As medicine evolves, new niches of expertise emerge, requiring specialist consultants.
  - *Contribution to health policy*: Using its expertise to influence policy and practice at national or international level.

The nurse researcher or consultant plays a crucial role by combining in-depth clinical expertise with a broad vision of healthcare. By tackling challenges with an evidence-based approach, they help shape the future of nursing and improve the quality of care for all patients.

Skills
and additional training
for career progression

The world of healthcare is constantly changing, and allergy and immunology nurses must constantly develop and adapt. Career progression often requires additional skills and training to meet the changing demands of the environment and to move into positions of greater responsibility or specialisation.

- Advanced training :
    - *Master's and PhD in Nursing*: These programmes offer in-depth training in research, leadership and education.
    - *Specialised certifications* : Certifications in Allergology, Immunology or other related fields can add formal recognition to specific expertise.
    - *Short courses and workshops*: These can cover new techniques, emerging technologies or specific topics such as medical ethics or stress management.
- Leadership and management skills :
    - *Team management*: Knowing how to motivate, lead and manage a team of nurses or healthcare professionals.
    - *Project management*: Planning, executing and evaluating care initiatives or research projects.
    - *Strategic decision-making*: Ability to see the big picture and make informed decisions for the good of the institution or department.
- Communication skills :
    - *Presentation and training*: Ability to teach, present lectures or conduct training courses.

- *Negotiation*: Knowing how to communicate effectively to obtain resources or collaborate with other departments.
- *Intercultural communication*: With the globalisation of healthcare, it is crucial to understand and interact effectively with people from different cultures.
- Technological skills :
  - *Medical informatics*: mastering health information systems, electronic medical records and related technologies.
  - *Telemedicine*: Understanding and effectively using remote care technologies, especially with the development of remote consultations.
  - *Data analysis* : With the growing importance of data in healthcare, the ability to analyse and interpret data is essential.
- Personal development and well-being :
  - *Stress management*: Learning techniques for managing the stress inherent in the profession.
  - *Resilience skills*: Ability to bounce back from trials or challenges.
  - *Networking*: Establish professional relationships within and outside your specialism to broaden your horizons and seize new opportunities.

Career progression for a nurse in Allergology and Immunology is not limited to mastering clinical skills. It encompasses a diverse range of interpersonal, technological and managerial skills. By continually investing in professional development and seeking out educational opportunities, the nurse can not only excel in their current role, but also pave the way for broader leadership opportunities and impact in the healthcare world.

Chapter 13:
REVIEW AND OUTLOOK

Where do Allergology and Immunology stand today?

Allergology and immunology, two closely related disciplines, have undergone major advances in recent decades, and their importance has increased in today's medical context. They are at the forefront of modern medicine, responding to complex health challenges and growing needs for specialist care.

- Increase in allergy cases:
  - In the industrialised world, we are witnessing a significant increase in allergic diseases. Respiratory, food and skin allergies have become more common, and studies suggest that environmental factors, lifestyle and even gut microbiota may play a role in this trend.
- Developments in immunological understanding :
  - The modern era of immunology has seen remarkable discoveries concerning the functioning of the immune system. Research into T and B cells, cytokines and the mechanisms of autoimmunity has led to a better understanding of immunological diseases.
- Advanced immunotherapies :
  - The development of innovative treatments, such as CAR-T therapies for certain cancers or immune checkpoint inhibitors, has revolutionised the treatment of diseases previously considered incurable.

- Personalised treatment :
  - Thanks to the era of genomic medicine, treatments can be tailored to the genetics and immunological profile of each patient, offering more targeted and effective approaches.
- Interconnection with other specialities :
  - Allergology and immunology have ramifications in other medical fields, such as dermatology, pneumology, gastroenterology and rheumatology, to name but a few. This convergence enables multidisciplinary therapeutic approaches.
- Persistent challenges :
  - Despite these advances, challenges remain. The growing prevalence of allergies and autoimmune diseases, associated with environmental and genetic factors, requires constant research to understand these phenomena.
- Impact of the COVID-19 pandemic :
  - The pandemic has highlighted the crucial importance of immunology. Understanding the immune response to the virus, developing vaccines in record time, and managing the immunological complications associated with the disease have reinforced the importance of this speciality.
- Emerging technologies :
  - The integration of artificial intelligence, bioinformatics and next-generation sequencing technologies promises to revolutionise the way we understand and treat allergic and immunological diseases.
- Education and awareness :
  - It has become imperative to educate the general public about allergies, the importance of vaccinations and understanding

immunological mechanisms in order to combat misinformation and promote prevention.

Allergology and Immunology are at an exciting crossroads, combining cutting-edge science, innovative treatments and growing clinical importance. With the rapid evolution of science and technology, the future of these disciplines is promising, although it is also fraught with challenges that will require perseverance, innovation and collaboration.

Future challenges for the speciality and for nurses

Allergology and immunology, like most medical disciplines, are constantly evolving. These specialities are at the heart of numerous debates and medical discoveries, and face significant challenges for the future. As an essential link in the healthcare chain, nurses will be directly affected and will need to adapt to these challenges.

- Increasing care for allergies :
  - With the worldwide increase in allergy cases, the demand for specialists and nurses trained in allergology will continue to grow. This means a greater workload, but also the need for ongoing training to keep up to date.
- Technological developments :
  - Technology is transforming medicine. The adoption of telemedicine, virtual reality for patient education and mobile applications for monitoring treatment are all elements that nurses will have to get used to.
- Complexity of new treatments :
  - With the advent of gene therapies, biotechnologies and sophisticated immunotherapies, nurses will need to

117

understand these treatments in depth in order to administer them safely and educate patients.

- Education and prevention :
    - The importance of preventing allergies and autoimmune diseases will require nurses to play an increasing role in educating patients and the general public.
- Interdisciplinary collaboration :
    - With Allergology and Immunology becoming increasingly interconnected with other specialties, nurses will need to work closely with professionals from other disciplines, requiring communication and coordination skills.
- Ethics and informed consent :
    - Future treatments, particularly those that genetically   modify the patient's own cells, will raise ethical issues. Nurses will need to be trained to discuss these issues with patients and obtain informed consent.
- Clinical research :
    - The importance of research in the development of the specialty cannot be underestimated. Nurses could play a more active role, not only by administering experimental treatments, but also by participating in the design and implementation of clinical studies.
- Global and environmental challenges:
    - Climate change, pollution and other environmental challenges are influencing the incidence of allergic and auto-immune diseases. Nurses need to be aware of these factors in order to adapt their care and advice.
- Emotional and psychological   support:
    - Patients with severe allergies or autoimmune diseases can face significant emotional

challenges. Nurses will need to strengthen their psychological support skills.
- Continuing education :
  - Given the rapid changes taking place in medicine, continuing training will be essential to ensure that nurses remain competent and up to date.

Allergology and Immunology, like any rapidly evolving medical field, offer both opportunities and challenges for nurses. By anticipating these issues and adapting proactively, nurses can ensure optimal care for their patients while enhancing their own careers.

Integrating new technologies and approaches

At the intersection of science, medicine and technology, Allergology and Immunology have witnessed an unprecedented transformation. Nurses, being at the forefront of patient care, play a central role in the integration and adoption of these advances. Understanding how these new technologies and approaches are shaping daily practice is essential for optimal patient care.

- Telemedicine and remote consultations :
  - **Definition**: Use of communication technologies to provide remote care.
  - **Applications in Allergology and Immunology**: patient monitoring, remote test interpretation, education and advice.
  - **Benefits**: Flexibility, accessibility for remote patients, reduced costs.
  - **Challenges**: Confidentiality, quality of patient-caregiver interaction, technical limitations.

- Mobile applications and handheld devices :
    - **Real-time monitoring**: Devices that monitor and record physiological parameters, such as oxygen levels, heart rate or allergic triggers.
    - **Adherence to treatment**: Applications reminding people to take their medication, following diets or action plans for seizures.
    - **Education and information**: Apps providing up-to-date information on allergies, pollen alerts or new discoveries in immunology.
- Augmented and virtual reality:
    - **Training and education**: Simulation of clinical situations to train nurses or educate patients.
    - **Guidance for procedures**: Used in real time to guide certain procedures or tests.
- Artificial Intelligence (AI) and Machine Learning:
    - **Assisted diagnosis**: Analysis of symptoms, clinical data and test results to suggest potential diagnoses.
    - **Personalised treatment**: AI can help predict a patient's response to a specific treatment or anticipate side effects.
- Genomics and personalised medicine :
    - **Genetic testing**: to identify genetic predispositions to allergies or autoimmune diseases.
    - **Targeted treatment**: Tailor treatments to the patient's genetic profile.
- Collaborative and interdisciplinary approaches :
    - **Online platforms**: Facilitating communication between specialists, nurses, GPs and other healthcare professionals.
    - **Centralised databases**: Gathering and analysing patient data to improve treatment and follow-up protocols.

- Training and updates :
    - **E-learning**: Use of online platforms for the continuing education of nurses.
    - **Webinars and virtual conferences**: Access the latest research and discussions in the field without being physically present.

New technologies and approaches offer promising solutions, but they require appropriate training and ethical reflection. For nurses, they offer the opportunity to improve the quality of care, optimise time and enhance their professional skills.

Advice for nurses who are starting their career in this speciality

Venturing into the specialist field of Allergology and Immunology may seem daunting at first, but it's an exciting opportunity to expand your knowledge, diversify your skills and make a significant impact on patients' lives. Here's some advice for those starting out on their journey:

- Continuing education :
    - **Regular updates**: The world of allergy and immunology is changing fast. Make sure you keep up to date with the latest advances and recommendations.
    - **Workshops and conferences**: Take part in specific training courses to enhance your practical skills.
- Mentoring :
    - **Find a mentor**: benefiting from the experience of a senior nurse can be invaluable.

She can guide you, answer your questions and offer moral support.

- Professional network :
  - **Joining associations** : Professional associations can offer opportunities for training, networking and access to valuable resources.
  - **Talk to your peers**: Talking to other nurses can help you share experiences, tips and advice.
- Patient-centred approach :
  - **Develop your communication skills**: active listening, empathy and the ability to explain medical information clearly are essential.
  - **Patient education**: Learn how to educate your patients about their condition, treatments and prevention.
- Stress management :
  - **Take care of yourself**: Burnout is real. Learn to recognise the signs and take breaks when you need to.
  - **Ask for help**: If you're feeling overwhelmed, talk to a supervisor or mentor.
- Organisation and efficiency :
  - **Time management**: With the number of patients and responsibilities, it's crucial to manage your time well.
  - **Accurate documentation**: Make sure that all care and interactions are accurately and exhaustively documented.
- Professional ethics :
  - **Confidentiality**: Always respect patient confidentiality.
  - **Integrity**: Always act in the patient's best interests and in accordance with medical guidelines.

- Adaptability :
  - **Embrace technology**: With the advent of new technologies, it's essential to be flexible and learn to use new tools.
- Long-term   outlook :
  - **Plan your career**: Think about where you want to be in 5, 10 or 15 years' time. Consider other training or specialisations if you are interested.
- Passion and dedication:
  - **Remember your motivation**: Difficult days will come, but remembering why you chose this path can help you persevere.

By starting out with determination, an open mind and a thirst for learning, allergy and immunology nurses can thrive in a career that is both rewarding and impactful.

Chapter 14:
INTERACTION WITH
OTHER MEDICAL SPECIALITIES

Collaboration with Dermatology

Allergology and Immunology share a fascinating interface with Dermatology, especially when considering skin diseases of allergic or immunological origin. This multidisciplinary interaction is not only crucial for accurate diagnosis, but also for providing integrated and comprehensive patient care.

- Intersections of specialities :
    - **Etiology of skin disorders** : Many skin conditions, such as eczema, urticaria and psoriasis, have an allergic or immunological component. Understanding these links can facilitate diagnosis and treatment.
    - **Skin manifestations of systemic allergies**: Some food or drug allergies can cause dermatological symptoms.
- The role of the allergy and immunology nurse :
    - **Interpretation of skin tests**: The nurse is often involved in the administration and interpretation of skin tests, and must therefore work closely with dermatologists.
    - **Patient education**: Inform patients about the links between their skin symptoms and possible allergies or immune imbalances.
- Collaboration in diagnosis :
    - **Sharing information**: Allergists and immunologists can provide valuable information about a patient's allergic history,

helping dermatologists to identify a possible aetiology.

- **Dermatoses of immune origin**: Diseases such as systemic lupus erythematosus and scleroderma require joint expertise in dermatology and immunology.
- Joint processing :
    - **Topical and systemic therapies**: For some conditions, both topical (dermatological) and systemic (allergological or immunological) treatment may be required.
    - **Monitoring side effects**: Some immunosuppressive treatments used in dermatology require immunological monitoring.
- Case studies and reviews :
    - **Multidisciplinary meetings**: Complex cases may benefit from joint meetings to discuss the best management strategies.
    - **Exchanges on the latest research**: advances in one area can influence practices in another.
- Training and awareness :
    - **Joint training programmes**: Workshops or training courses can be organised jointly to provide better information on the intersections between the two specialities.
    - **Raising public awareness**: Informing the public about the links between allergies, immunology and skin disorders.
- Future prospects :
    - **Collaborative research**: Interdisciplinary research can lead to new discoveries and improvements in the treatment of skin conditions of allergic or immunological origin.
    - **Development of combined therapies**: The future could see the development of treatments

that combine expertise in allergology, immunology and dermatology.

Close collaboration between Allergology, Immunology and Dermatology is not only desirable but often necessary to ensure holistic patient care. For the nurse, this collaboration translates into better understanding, better training and, ultimately, more comprehensive care for the patient.

Interactions with Respirology

Allergology and Immunology have close links with Respirology, as many respiratory diseases have an allergic or immunological origin. Understanding these interactions is vital for diagnosing, treating and managing associated lung diseases.

- Intersections of specialities :
  - **Origin of respiratory diseases**: Diseases such as asthma, allergic bronchitis and certain pneumonias have clear allergic or immunological components.
  - **Respiratory manifestations of immunological disorders**: Certain immune diseases can have pulmonary consequences, as in the case of sarcoidosis.
- The role of the allergy and immunology nurse :
  - **Interpretation of pulmonary function tests**: Nurses often play a role in the administration of tests such as spirometry, and must therefore work closely with pulmonologists.
  - **Patient education**: Patients should be informed of the links between their respiratory symptoms and possible allergies or immune imbalances.

- Collaboration in diagnosis :
  - **Sharing information**: Allergists and immunologists can offer valuable information about a patient's allergic history, enlightening pulmonologists about a potential aetiology.
  - **Lung diseases of immune origin**: The management of diseases such as interstitial pneumonia linked to an autoimmune disease requires expertise in both pneumology and immunology.
- Joint processing :
  - **Inhaled and systemic therapies**: Diseases such as asthma may require a combination of inhaled and systemic treatments.
  - **Monitoring for side effects**: Certain immunomodulatory treatments used for lung diseases may require immunological monitoring.
- Case studies and reviews :
  - **Multidisciplinary meetings**: Complex cases can benefit from joint discussions to develop the best management strategies.
  - **Exchanges on the latest research**: advances in one field can directly influence practices in another.
- Training and awareness :
  - **Joint training programmes**: Seminars or workshops can be organised to enhance the cross-fertilisation of knowledge between pulmonology and allergology-immunology.
  - **Raising public awareness**: educating the public about the relationship between allergies, immunology and lung diseases.
- Future prospects :
  - **Collaborative research**: Joint research can lead to new methods for diagnosing or treating

respiratory diseases linked to allergies or immune disorders.

- **Innovative therapies**: Future therapies could benefit from the combined expertise of pulmonologists, allergists and immunologists.

The symbiosis between Respirology, Allergology and Immunology is fundamental to optimal patient care. The nurse, at the crossroads of these specialities, is an essential link, facilitating communication and the coordination of care between the various medical players.

Working with Gastroenterology for food allergies

Food allergy is an area where allergy and gastroenterology intersect closely. The symptoms of a food allergy can manifest themselves both in the digestive system and at other levels of the body. Collaboration between allergists, immunologists and gastroenterologists is therefore essential if patients are to be treated comprehensively.

- Background to food allergies :
    - **Symptoms**: The symptoms of a food allergy can be varied, ranging from simple itching in the mouth to digestive problems and even anaphylactic shock.
    - **Frequency**: With an increase in cases of food allergy, the need for a multidisciplinary approach has become more pressing.
- Joint diagnosis :
    - **Detailed history**: The nurse plays a crucial role in gathering accurate information about the patient's eating habits and associated symptoms.

- **Allergy tests**: carried out by the allergist to determine specific allergens.
- **Gastroenterological examinations**: carried out by the gastroenterologist to identify and assess any damage or inflammation of the digestive system.
- Collaborative processing strategies :
    - **Avoidance**: Avoiding the allergen in question is often the first step in treatment.
    - **Medication**: Antihistamines, corticoids or others to treat symptoms. In the case of severe digestive disorders, specific gastroenterological treatments may be necessary.
    - **Therapeutic education**: Patients need to learn how to recognise and avoid potentially dangerous foods, as well as how to manage emergency situations.
- Interdisciplinary approaches :
    - **Joint case studies**: Discussion of complex cases between specialists to develop optimal management strategies.
    - **Research and studies**: Collaborating on clinical studies or research to better understand the mechanisms of food allergies and develop new treatment methods.
- The importance of communication :
    - **Information sharing**: Ensure smooth communication between allergists, gastroenterologists and nurses to ensure that all patient concerns are addressed.
    - **Care coordination**: As care coordinator, the nurse ensures that the patient receives holistic care.
- Continuing education :
    - **Joint education**: Training and workshops for professionals can help them better understand

the complexities of food allergies and their gastrointestinal manifestations.
- **Knowledge update**: With advances in research, approaches to treatment are evolving.
- Future prospects :
  - **Innovative therapies**: As research progresses, new treatments for food allergies could emerge, requiring close collaboration between specialities for their implementation.

The link between allergy and gastroenterology in the context of food allergies is undeniable. Nurses, with their central role in coordination and communication, are essential in guaranteeing effective and comprehensive care for patients affected by these allergies.

Allergology and Immunology in paediatric settings

The care of children with allergic and immunological disorders presents specific challenges and nuances. Children are not simply "little adults"; their immune systems are still developing, their eating habits differ, and their environments (particularly schools) impose particular constraints.

- Pediatric specificities :
  - **Developing immune system**: In children, the immune system is still maturing, sometimes making diagnosis and treatment more difficult.
  - **Different clinical presentation**: The symptoms of allergies and immune disorders can vary depending on the age of the patient.

- Common allergies in children :
  - **Food allergies**: Allergies to milk, eggs, peanuts and others.
  - **Respiratory allergies**: Asthma, allergic rhinitis linked in particular to house dust mites or pollen.
  - **Atopic eczema: A** common skin condition in young children.
- Tests and diagnostics specific to paediatrics :
  - **Adaptation of skin tests**: Take into account the sensitivity of children's skin.
  - **Interpretation of blood tests**: Normal values may differ according to age.
- Therapeutic   approaches :
  - **Medicines** : Adapting dosages, taking paediatric forms into account.
  - **Immunotherapy**: Determining the appropriate age to start, close monitoring of side effects.
  - **Therapeutic education**: adapting information to the child's age, involving the family.
- Psychosocial challenges :
  - **Adapting to school**: Working with schools to ensure children's safety (food allergies, asthma).
  - **Psychological support**: Helping children to manage the fear, anxiety and stigma associated with their condition.
- Working with the family :
  - **Parent education**: Providing resources and training to help parents manage their child's condition on a daily basis.
  - **Emergency action plan**: Ensure that parents, carers and teachers are well informed and equipped.

- Transition to adult care :
    - **Preparation and education**: Preparing teenagers to manage their condition independently.
    - **Coordination with adult services**: Ensuring a smooth transition to another specialist when the child reaches adulthood.
- Research and the future :
    - **Paediatric studies**: Emphasise the importance of research specific to the paediatric population.
    - **New treatments and approaches**: Monitoring advances in research to offer children the best treatment options.

Paediatric allergology and immunology require an in-depth understanding of the specific characteristics of children and close collaboration with their family and school environment. The nurse plays a crucial role in this care, acting as a liaison between doctors, parents, educators and, of course, the young patients themselves.

Chapter 15:
NUTRITIONAL ASPECTS
IN ALLERGOLOGY

The impact of nutrition
on the immune system

Nutrition plays an essential role in maintaining health and well-being. It influences many aspects of human physiology, including the immune system. Adequate nutrition can strengthen the body's natural defences, while malnutrition can weaken them, making the individual more susceptible to infections and other ailments.

- Fundamental principles of nutrition :
    - **Macronutrients** : Proteins, fats, carbohydrates - their role and importance.
    - **Micronutrients** : Vitamins and minerals essential for optimal functioning of the immune system.
- Immunity and nutrition :
    - **Supporting innate immunity**: How nutrition influences physical barriers such as the skin and mucous membranes.
    - **Support for adaptive immunity**: The role of nutrients in the proliferation and function of T and B cells.
- Key vitamins and minerals for immunity :
    - **Vitamin C**: Importance for immune cell health, dietary sources and recommendations.
    - **Vitamin D**: Role in modulating innate and adaptive immunity, sources and recommendations.

- **Zinc**: Support for immune cell function, signs of deficiency, and dietary sources.
- **Selenium, iron, copper**: Their role in immunity and how to incorporate them into the diet.
- Beneficial foods and compounds :
  - **Probiotics and prebiotics**: their role in supporting intestinal health and immunity.
  - **Antioxidants** : How they protect cells against oxidative damage.
  - **Anti-inflammatory foods**: The benefits of omega-3, turmeric and other compounds.
- Malnutrition and immunity :
  - **Effects of malnutrition**: How inadequate nutritional intake weakens the immune system.
  - **At-risk groups**: Children, the elderly, people with chronic illnesses.
- Specific diets and immunity :
  - **Mediterranean, vegetarian, ketogenic diet**: Benefits and precautions for immune health.
- Drug interactions and nutrition :
  - **Immunosuppressive drugs**: how they can affect nutritional requirements.
  - Drug-food interactions: What to watch out for and what to avoid.

- Practical advice for a stronger immune system :
  - **Meal planning**: Include nutrient-rich foods to support immunity.
  - **Supplements** : When are they needed? Precautions to take.

Understanding the relationship between nutrition and immunity is crucial for anyone working in the medical field. A balanced, nutrient-rich diet is one of the keys to maintaining a robust immune system, helping to prevent illness and promote rapid recovery when it does occur. For Allergy and Immunology nurses, this knowledge can be particularly relevant when providing therapeutic patient education.

Dietetics for allergy sufferers

Food allergy is an adverse reaction of the immune system to a food or food component, usually a protein. Dietary management of allergic patients is fundamental to preventing reactions, ensuring adequate growth and development, and maintaining a satisfactory quality of life. For allergy nurses, having a basic knowledge of dietetics can be invaluable in educating and supporting patients.

- Understanding common food allergens:
    - **The "Big Eight"**: The eight major allergens that cause the majority of allergic reactions: milk, eggs, peanuts, nuts, soya, wheat, fish and shellfish.
    - **Other allergens**: Sesame seeds, mustard, sulphites and others.
- Diagnosing a food allergy:
    - **Common symptoms**: Urticaria, oedema, gastrointestinal disorders, anaphylaxis.
    - **Diagnostic tests**: skin tests, blood tests, avoidance diet.
- Dietary   advice to avoid allergens:
    - **Reading labels**: Identify potentially allergenic ingredients.
    - **Food preparation**: Avoid cross-contamination at home.
    - **Eating out**: Questions to ask the restaurant, beware of buffets.
- Food substitutes for common allergens:
    - **Dairy substitutes**: Plant-based milks, lactose-free products.

- **Egg substitutes**: Apple sauce, silken tofu, commercial mixes.
- **Gluten substitutes**: Gluten-free flours, xanthan and guar gum.
- Nutritional management of multiple allergies:
  - **Meal planning**: Ensuring a balanced nutritional intake despite restrictions.
  - **Supplements**: When are they needed? Vitamins, minerals.
- Emotional and psychological support:
  - **Living with restrictions**: Acceptance, resilience, seeking support.
  - Support for children and their families: workshops, support groups, education.
- Awareness-raising and education:
  - **Raising awareness in the community**: family, school, workplace.
  - **Anaphylaxis education**: recognising symptoms, use of epipens, emergency action plan.
- Current trends and advances in food allergology:
  - **Emerging therapies**: Oral immunotherapy, exposure patches.
  - **Research and future hopes**: Towards a better understanding and more effective treatments.
- Resources and references for patients:
  - **Support organisations**: Food allergy associations.
  - **Online applications and tools**: Help with allergy management and education.

Allergy and Immunology nurses play an essential role in educating patients about allergy-related dietetics. Helping them to understand their allergies, avoid allergens and manage their reactions, while ensuring they receive adequate nutrition, is essential to their overall well-being.

Supplementation and immunotherapy

The interaction between nutrition, supplementation and the immune system is an exciting area of research. At the same time, immunotherapy, which modifies the immune response to treat or prevent disease, is revolutionising the treatment of allergies and other conditions. Allergology and Immunology nurses therefore need to be aware of the intersections between these two fields.

- The impact of nutrition on immunity:
    - **The role of nutrients**: How vitamins, minerals and other nutrients influence immune function.
    - **Nutritional deficiencies**: how they can weaken the immune system and increase susceptibility to disease.
- Supplements to support immunity:
    - **Vitamin C and Zinc**: Their role in strengthening the immune barrier.
    - **Probiotics**: How they can modulate the immune response and their potential use in allergies.
    - **Omega-3**: Natural anti-inflammatories and their impact on autoimmune and allergic conditions.
    - **Selection and safety**: How to choose a supplement and the precautions to take.
- Allergen immunotherapy:
    - **Basic principle**: gradually expose the patient to the allergen to induce tolerance.
    - **Types of immunotherapy**: Sublingual, subcutaneous, exposure patches.
    - **Patient selection**: Who could benefit from immunotherapy?

- Managing side effects and reactions:
    - **Common side effects**: Itching, swelling, more serious reactions.
    - **Monitoring and intervention**: The crucial role of the nurse in detecting and managing reactions.
- The future of immunotherapy:
    - **New targets**: Beyond common allergens, treatments for severe food allergies.
    - **Personalised approaches**: Adapting treatments based on genetic and environmental factors.
- Supplementation during immunotherapy:
    - **Potential interactions**: How certain supplements might affect the efficacy of immunotherapy.
    - **Supporting the immune system**: Supplements that might enhance the benefits of immunotherapy.
- The nurse's educational role:
    - **Patient education**: Inform patients about immunotherapy, its benefits and risks, and the importance of adequate supplementation.
    - **Raising public awareness**: Promoting a better understanding of immunotherapy and nutrition as tools in the management of allergies.

The combination of appropriate supplementation and immunotherapy can offer a holistic approach to the management of allergies and other immune conditions. Allergy and Immunology nurses are at the forefront of helping patients navigate these treatments, providing information, support and specialist care.

The influence of current diets on allergies

Dietary habits and trends have undergone many changes over the decades. These changes, in combination with other factors, can have an impact on the incidence and severity of allergies. Understanding this relationship is crucial for allergy and immunology nurses, as it offers insights into the prevention and management of food allergies.

- The evolution of diets:
    - **Modern industrial diets**: Increased consumption of processed foods, additives, preservatives and chemicals.
    - **Fashionable diets**: From gluten-free to vegan, via the paleo diet and the ketogenic diet.
- Food additives and allergies:
    - **Dyes and preservatives**: their potential role in sensitisation and allergenic reactivity.
    - **Emulsifiers and stabilisers**: How they can affect the intestinal barrier and potentially contribute to allergic reactions.
- Excessive hygiene and the intestinal microbiota:
    - **Hygiene theory**: How living in environments that are too clean could contribute to an increase in allergies.
    - **Impact of diet on the microbiota**: How the foods we eat influence intestinal bacteria and, consequently, our immune response.
- Allergies and elimination diets:
    - **Gluten-free diet**: Impacts on intestinal health and wheat sensitivity.
    - **Dairy-free diets**: their effects on lactose tolerance and milk protein allergies.
- Nutritional deficiencies and allergic sensitivity:
    - **Vitamin D**: Its potential role in modulating the immune response.

- **Omega-3**: How reduced consumption of omega-3 fatty acids in modern diets can contribute to allergic reactions.
- The nurse's educational role:
  - **Dietary advice for allergy sufferers**: educating on the importance of reading labels, recognising hidden allergens and understanding the implications of food choices.
  - **Promoting a balanced diet**: Encourage a diet rich in fruit, vegetables, whole grains and varied sources of protein to boost the immune system.
- Recommendations for patients:
  - **Food allergy tests**: When and how to do them, and their interpretation.
  - **Adapting the diet**: how to avoid allergens while ensuring a balanced, nutritious diet.

Ultimately, diet plays a crucial role in overall health and immune function. Allergy and Immunology nurses have a unique opportunity to educate and guide patients through the complexities of modern diets and their potential impact on allergies.

Chapter 16:
ALTERNATIVE APPROACHES AND COMPLEMENTARY

Traditional medicine in the face of allergies and immune deficiencies

Traditional medicine's approach to allergies and immune deficiencies is a rich and varied mix of experiences, beliefs and therapeutic methods developed over centuries. From traditional Chinese medicine to Indian Ayurveda, these systems offer complementary perspectives, sometimes used in tandem with modern medicine.

- Origins and philosophies:
    - **Traditional Chinese medicine (TCM)**: Based on the concept of balance between Yin and Yang and the circulation of Qi (vital energy).
    - **Ayurveda:** The ancient Indian medical system based on balancing the three doshas: vata, pitta and kapha.
    - **Traditional African medicine**: The importance of ancestors, spirits and medicinal herbs.
    - **Western phytotherapy**: Use of medicinal plants based on experience and tradition.
- Diagnostic approaches:
    - **Pulse and tongue in TCM**: How palpation of the pulse and examination of the tongue can indicate energy imbalances.
    - **Diagnosis by observation in Ayurveda**: Examine the skin, eyes, nails and other

physical signs to determine the dominant dosha and imbalances.

- Traditional allergy treatments:
    - **Acupuncture and moxibustion**: The use of fine needles and heat to rebalance Qi and treat allergic symptoms.
    - **Herbs and remedies**: Like quercetin, turmeric and other medicinal plants with anti-inflammatory and antihistaminic properties.
    - **Breathing techniques and meditation**: Helps to relax and reduce stress, often used in Ayurveda.
    - **Massages and body therapies**: To stimulate circulation and facilitate detoxification.
- Management of immune deficiencies:
    - **Tonics and adaptogens**: Herbs such as ginseng, ashwagandha or astragalus root to boost immunity.
    - **Traditional dietetics**: Foods recommended for boosting the immune system, such as chicken soup, bone broth or fermented foods.
    - **Spiritual practices and rituals**: Prayers, meditations or rituals to balance mind and body.
- Limits and interactions:
    - **Drug interactions**: It is important to be aware of potential interactions between traditional remedies and modern medicines.
    - **Research and evidence**: While some traditional methods are supported by modern research, others require further study.
- The allergy and immunology nurse and traditional medicine:
    - **Open communication**: Encouraging patients to share the traditional remedies they use.

- **Continuing education**: Keeping abreast of the latest research into traditional treatments and their effectiveness.

By embracing the richness of traditional medicine while respecting the principles of modern medicine, Allergy and Immunology nurses can offer holistic, patient-centred care, addressing both physical and emotional needs.

Homeopathy and Allergology

Homeopathy, a branch of alternative medicine that originated in the 18th century, is based on the principle of "similia similibus curentur" or "like cures like". In allergy, this approach is of some interest, as allergic symptoms are often the result of the body's reaction to substances which, in higher concentrations, could cause similar symptoms in a healthy person.

- Foundations of homeopathy:
    - **The law of similars**: The philosophical basis underlying the principle that substances which cause symptoms in a healthy person can, in infinitesimal doses, cure similar symptoms in a sick person.
    - **Dilution and dynamisation**: The unique process of preparing homeopathic remedies, where the original substance is sequentially diluted and vigorously shaken or "dynamised".
- Homeopathy in the treatment of allergies:
    - **Allium cepa**: Often used to treat hay fever symptoms similar to those caused by exposure to onions, such as watery eyes.
    - **Apis mellifica: For** allergic reactions that resemble bee stings, with swelling and itching.
    - **Euphrasia:** For allergy-prone eye symptoms.

143

- Studies and efficiency:
  - **Current research**: Although some studies suggest that homeopathy could be effective for certain allergic conditions, the methodology and results often remain controversial.
  - **Placebo and the effect of homeopathy**: Discussion of the frequent argument that the effect of homeopathy may be mainly placebo.
- Nurses and homeopathy:
  - **Listening and openness**: It is essential to listen to patients who choose to follow a homeopathic treatment and to inform them of the benefits and limitations.
  - **Interactions and integration**: Make sure that homeopathic treatments do not contradict other medical treatments.
- Current criticisms and debates:
  - **Scientific scepticism**: Many experts believe that homeopathy does not go beyond the placebo effect due to the high dilution of the remedies.
  - **Defenders of homeopathy**: They claim that the mechanisms of action of homeopathy are not yet fully understood, but that they offer a real benefit to many patients.
- Conclusion and the future of homeopathy in allergy:
  - The changing perception and acceptance of homeopathy.
  - The need for more robust and systematic studies to shed light on its role in the treatment of allergies.

Homeopathy in allergy is a complex field that combines tradition, philosophy and science. It is crucial that allergy and immunology nurses are well-informed and open to this approach in order to offer integrative, patient-centred care.

Naturopathic approaches and nutrition

Naturopathy, a traditional, holistic medicine, offers complementary tools for preventing and treating allergies and immune disorders. It considers the patient as a whole, integrating the physical, mental and environmental aspects. The emphasis is on natural approaches, particularly nutritional ones, to strengthen the immune system and treat imbalances.

- Foundations of naturopathy:
    - **Basic principles**: The philosophy of naturopathy aims to stimulate the body's self-healing capacity, with an emphasis on prevention.
    - **The six pillars**: lifestyle, diet, psychology, hydrology, phytology and manual techniques.
- Nutrition and allergies:
    - **The role of food**: Understanding how what we eat can affect our immune system and our allergic reactions.
    - **Anti-inflammatory foods**: The benefits of omega-3s, antioxidants and other key nutrients in moderating allergic responses.
- Managing allergies through nutrition:
    - **Elimination and rotation**: Techniques for identifying and managing food allergies.
    - **Probiotics and gut health**: The importance of a healthy microbiome in modulating the immune response.
- Plants and supplements in Allergology:
    - **Quercetin, nettle and others**: Their potential roles in reducing allergic symptoms.

- **Vitamin C and bioflavonoids**: How they can support immune function and modulate the allergic reaction.
- Nurses and naturopathic approaches:
    - **Information and advice**: Helping patients to navigate the vast world of natural remedies.
    - **Interaction and integration**: Ensuring a coherent and safe approach between conventional and naturopathic treatments.
- Challenges and criticism:
    - **Lack of robust studies**: The need for more in-depth research into the effectiveness of naturopathic interventions.
    - **Potential risks**: Although natural, some remedies may present risks of interactions or side effects.
- Conclusion and future prospects:
    - **Increasing integration**: With increasing demand for integrative care, Allergology and Immunology could see greater integration of naturopathic approaches.
    - **Continuing education for healthcare professionals**: The need for training to understand, advise on and integrate these approaches into clinical practice.

The world of naturopathy offers a range of tools that can complement traditional treatments in allergy and immunology. Nurses can play a pivotal role in informing, guiding and supporting their patients as they explore these complementary methods.

Effectiveness, risks and recommendations

Medical practice is constantly evolving with the arrival of new data, therapies and technologies. In allergy and immunology, treatments must be based on solid scientific evidence. However, the growing demand for integrative and complementary approaches requires rigorous evaluation of their efficacy and safety.

- Evaluation of effectiveness:
    - **The importance of clinical trials**: how they provide a solid basis for assessing the effectiveness of treatments.
    - **Meta-analyses and systematic reviews**: The importance of pooling data to obtain more robust conclusions.
- Risks associated with treatment:
    - **Common side effects**: Identifying and managing adverse reactions in Allergology and Immunology.
    - **Drug interactions**: The need to monitor interactions, especially with the introduction of complementary therapies.
- Evidence-based clinical recommendations:
    - **Guidelines**: How clinical recommendations are drawn up and their importance in everyday practice.
    - **The importance of constant updating**: Ensure that recommendations reflect the latest discoveries and standards of excellence.
- Complementary and integrative approaches:
    - **Effectiveness and safety**: Evaluation of alternative therapies such as naturopathy, homeopathy and others.

- **Integration into clinical practice**: How and when to incorporate these methods safely.
- The patient's perspective:
  - **Patient autonomy and informed consent**: Inform the patient of the benefits and risks associated with each treatment.
  - **Understanding patient preferences and beliefs**: The role of cultural and personal beliefs in the choice of treatment.
- Training and skills for healthcare professionals:
  - **Continuous updating of knowledge**: The importance of ongoing training to stay at the cutting edge of advances in Allergology and Immunology.
  - **Communication skills**: How to effectively discuss treatment options, risks and benefits with patients.
- Conclusion and future prospects:
  - **The future of Allergology and Immunology**: The potential impact of new discoveries and technologies on the efficacy and safety of treatments.
  - **Ethics and integrity in practice**: Ensuring that treatments are always based on solid evidence, while respecting patients' wishes and rights.

The balance between efficacy and risk is at the heart of medical practice. In Allergology and Immunology, it is essential that nurses are well informed, not only about conventional treatments, but also about complementary approaches, in order to provide integrated, evidence-based care to their patients.

Chapter 17:
ENVIRONMENTAL ISSUES AND ALLERGOLOGY

Impact of pollution on the increase in allergies

The worldwide rise in allergic diseases is a growing concern for health professionals and society as a whole. One of the main theories behind this surge is the impact of pollution on respiratory and immunological health. Understanding this impact not only helps to raise awareness of the seriousness of the problem, but also to develop more effective preventive and therapeutic strategies.

- Introduction:
    - **Current statistics**: Allergy cases have been on the rise for decades.
    - Links between urbanisation, industrialisation and allergies: A global overview of the problem.
- Air pollutants and their sources:
    - **Primary and secondary pollutants**: Understanding the difference and where they come from.
    - **Industrial emissions, transport and agriculture**: How do these sectors contribute to air pollution?
- Underlying biological mechanisms:
    - **Inflammatory reactions**: How pollutants can trigger or exacerbate allergic reactions.
    - **Changes to allergens**: Can pollution make certain allergens more reactive or virulent?

- Respiratory allergies:
  - **Asthma**: The impact of pollution on the prevalence and severity of asthma.
  - **Allergic rhinitis**: The correlation between pollution and hay fever symptoms.
- Skin and eye allergies:
  - **Eczema and urticaria**: How does pollution affect these conditions?
  - **Allergic conjunctivitis**: The effect of pollutants on the eyes.
- Long-term consequences:
  - **Increased sensitivity**: Can repeated exposure increase sensitivity to certain allergens?
  - **Associated complications**: The impact on other respiratory or systemic diseases.
- Preventive and therapeutic strategies:
  - **Avoiding and reducing exposure**: Practical advice for limiting the impact of pollution.
  - **Medicinal treatments**: Adapt treatments according to pollution levels.
- Public policy and environmental health:
  - **Air quality regulations**: The role of governments in limiting pollution.
  - **Raising public awareness**: Educating society about the associated risks and promoting more environmentally-friendly behaviour.
- Conclusion:
  - **The need for collective action**: Faced with a growing threat, it is essential to join forces to combat pollution and its effects on health.
  - The future of Allergology in a changing world: Reflections on the challenges and opportunities ahead.

Air pollution is a silent threat that has a major influence on the prevalence and severity of allergies. As allergy and immunology nurses, it is essential to be aware of this correlation, to understand its mechanisms and to take both clinical and preventive action.

Seasonal allergies and climate change

Climate change, with its changes in temperature and weather patterns, has direct consequences for human health. Of particular concern is the impact on seasonal allergies. Flowering periods are lengthening, pollen concentrations are increasing, and regions traditionally free of certain allergens are beginning to show signs of them. Allergy and immunology healthcare professionals are on the front line in understanding and treating these new realities.

- Introduction:
    - Definition of seasonal allergies: A reminder of what they encompass.
    - **Climate change**: How our planet is changing and why it matters.
- Impact of temperature on allergens:
    - **Longer pollen seasons**: How global warming is extending the flowering period of allergenic plants.
    - Increased pollen concentrations: more CO_2, more pollen.
- Allergen migration:
    - **New territories**: Allergenic plants are now establishing themselves in previously unaffected areas.
    - **Allergens at altitude**: Mountains are no longer refuges.

- Impact on public health:
  - **Increase in prevalence**: More people are allergic than ever before.
  - **Worsening of symptoms**: Reactions may be more intense.
- Changes in exposure patterns:
  - **Multiple exposure**: The coexistence of different allergens in a single season.
  - **Extreme weather**: how pollen storms and other phenomena affect patients.
- Adaptation strategies for healthcare professionals:
  - **Updating protocols**: adapting tests and treatments to new allergens.
  - **Therapeutic patient education**: Informing patients about new risks and how to manage them.
- Prevention and monitoring:
  - **Pollen monitoring**: Using technology to predict and provide information on pollen concentrations.
  - **Advice for patients**: How to avoid exposure during pollen peaks.
- Research and innovation:
  - **Epidemiological studies**: Monitoring allergy trends on a global scale.
  - **Developing targeted treatments**: The importance of research in adapting to new challenges.
- Conclusion:
  - **A call to action**: The need for joint action by healthcare professionals, governments and civil society.
  - **The future of seasonal allergies**: Projections and preparations for the coming decades.

With climate change as a backdrop, Allergology and Immunology must evolve rapidly to meet the changing needs of patients. Nurses, as the key point of contact for many patients, have a crucial role to play in helping to navigate this changing reality.

Housing and household allergens

The home, a place of rest and security, can paradoxically become a source of exposure to numerous allergens. From house dust mites to mould and pet hair, the home is full of pitfalls for allergy sufferers. For allergy and immunology professionals, it is essential to understand their patients' home environment and advise them on how to minimise the risks.

- Introduction:
    - **The importance of the home in health**: How the domestic environment influences health.
    - **Definition of household allergens**: Presentation of the main culprits.
- Mites:
    - **Biology and favourite habitats**: Where and why they thrive.
    - Associated symptoms and diagnoses.
    - **Prevention and control strategies**: from anti-dust mite bedding to appropriate hygrometry.
- Animal hair and dander:
    - **Commonly associated animals**: Dogs, cats, birds, etc.
    - Recognising and managing an allergy: Tests and symptoms.
    - **Living with pets**: Tips for minimising exposure.

- Mould and fungi:
  - **Where can they be found?** Damp areas, cellars, bathrooms, etc.
  - Associated health problems.
  - **Home prevention and treatment**: Ventilation, dehumidifiers, anti-mould products.
- Allergens in the kitchen:
  - **Insects and pests**: Cockroaches and other common insects.
  - **Food storage** : How to avoid infestations and associated allergens.
- Household products and allergies:
  - **Common irritant compounds**: Perfumes, detergents, disinfectants.
  - **Selecting and using safe products**: Opt for hypoallergenic products, read labels.
- Indoor plants and allergies:
  - Commonly allergenic plants.
  - **Benefits of plants for air quality**: How certain plants can purify the air.
- Home improvements for allergy sufferers:
  - **Materials and furniture**: Choose non-allergenic materials.
  - **Ventilation and air filtration**: Purification systems, HEPA filters.
- General preventive measures:
  - **Cleaning routine**: Frequency, tools and appropriate techniques.
  - **Patient education**: The importance of information and awareness.
- Conclusion:
- **A suitable environment for everyone**: The importance of a healthy home for quality of life.
- **Role of the healthcare professional**: Accompanying, advising and educating patients.

Controlling household allergens is an essential part of allergy management. By understanding the patient's home and helping them to implement preventive measures, nurses can make a significant contribution to improving their quality of life.

Tips for healthy living
in an allergenic environment

In a world where allergens are ubiquitous, living a healthy and fulfilling life can seem like navigating through a minefield for those with sensitivities. However, with the right knowledge and a proactive attitude, it is entirely possible to lead a full life while effectively managing your allergies.

Here's a guide to help people live peacefully in an allergen-rich environment.

- Awareness and education:
    - **Understanding allergies**: the importance of allergy tests and regular check-ups.
    - **Keeping up to date**: Stay up to date on research, new treatments and seasonal forecasts.
- Healthy living:
    - **Choosing the right place to live**: looking for an area with fewer specific allergens.
    - **Air purifiers**: Invest in quality systems to filter out allergens.
    - **Regular maintenance**: Clean, vacuum and ventilate to reduce the presence of allergens.
- Conscious eating:
    - **Reading labels**: Avoid hidden allergens in processed products.

- **Home preparation**: Check ingredients and cooking methods.
- **Be vigilant in the restaurant**: Clearly communicate allergies to staff.
- Trips and outings:
  - **Prior research**: Check for the presence of potential allergens in the chosen destination.
  - **Emergency kit**: Always take emergency medicines and treatments with you.
  - **Adapted accommodation**: Look for hotels or accommodation that take allergies into account.
- Stress management:
  - **Link between stress and allergic symptoms**: Understanding how stress can exacerbate allergies.
  - **Relaxation techniques**: meditation, yoga, deep breathing to maintain emotional balance.
- An active, safe lifestyle:
  - **Sports and outdoor activities**: Choose times when allergen levels are low.
  - **Gyms and sports clubs**: Check air quality and cleanliness of facilities.
- Relationships and social life:
  - **Open communication**: telling friends and family about your allergies.
  - **Taking part in support groups**: sharing experiences and tips with other allergy sufferers.
- Career and working environment:
  - **Choose a healthy workplace**: Avoid confined or dusty spaces.
  - **Adapt your space**: Purifying plants, air purifiers and regular breaks to air out.

- Technology to the rescue:
    - **Applications and gadgets**: Using technological tools to monitor and manage allergies.
    - **Telemedicine**: consulting specialists at a distance, especially when travelling.
- Blossoming   in spite of everything:
- **Celebrate the small victories**: Acknowledge the symptom-free moments and the progress made.
- **Adopt a positive attitude**: Focus on what is possible rather than on restrictions.

With a well thought-out strategy, a healthy life in an allergenic environment is entirely achievable. It involves a combination of preparation, education and a proactive approach to minimising risks while maximising quality of life.

Chapter 18:
INFORMATION TECHNOLOGY
IN ALLERGOLOGY AND IMMUNOLOGY

Electronic medical records
and their usefulness

The electronic medical record (EMR) represents a major transformation in healthcare, changing the way professionals access, store and share patient information. Discussing its benefits and challenges, this section highlights the importance of EMRs in modern medical practice.

- What is an EMR?
    - **Definition**: An EMR is a digital record of a patient's health information.
    - **Evolution**: From paper to digital - understanding how the EMR was born out of the need to improve efficiency and accuracy.
- Advantages of EMR:
    - **Rapid access**: Data can be retrieved instantly, facilitating diagnosis and treatment.
    - **Simplified sharing**: healthcare professionals can share crucial information, promoting multidisciplinary care.
    - **Reduced errors**: Fewer errors due to misread handwriting or lost files.
    - **Optimised management**: monitoring vaccinations, reminders for screening tests, and prescription management.
- EMRs in Allergology and Immunology:
    - **Allergy test monitoring**: easily record and compare the results of skin or blood tests.

- **Treatment management**: Monitoring immunotherapy, biological treatments and associated side-effects.
- Security and confidentiality:
  - **Protecting sensitive data:** security mechanisms to prevent unauthorised access.
  - **Compliance with regulatory standards**: Ensuring compliance with privacy legislation.
- Integration with other systems:
  - **Interconnectivity**: Links with laboratories, pharmacies and other care facilities.
  - **Telemedicine**: Facilitating remote consultations by making data available online.
- Challenges and obstacles:
  - **Initial costs**: Investment in hardware, software and training.
  - **Resistance to change**: Adoption by staff may require a period of adaptation.
  - **Updates and maintenance: The** need for continuous technological monitoring.
- Training and skills:
  - **Learning to use the EMR**: Importance of training staff to use the system effectively.
  - **Optimising use**: making full use of functionality to improve care.
- The future of DME:
  - **Technological innovations**: artificial intelligence, machine learning and other advances.
  - **Standardisation**: Harmonisation of systems for greater interoperability at national and international level.

Electronic medical records have revolutionised the way care is delivered, offering speed, efficiency and accuracy. For Allergy and Immunology nurses, they are an invaluable tool, enabling patients to be followed in detail and guaranteeing the best possible quality of care.

Digital applications and platforms for patient monitoring

The advent of technology has profoundly transformed the medical landscape, particularly in the field of Allergology and Immunology. Dedicated applications and digital platforms now offer unprecedented possibilities for monitoring patients, making care more accessible, personalised and effective.

- Introduction to medical   applications:
    - **Definition and objectives**: To understand what a medical application is and how it can facilitate patient monitoring.
    - **Evolution and adoption**: How have apps gained in popularity and how are they being integrated into everyday medical practice?
- Allergy monitoring applications:
    - **Allergy diary**: Allows patients to record their symptoms, triggers and medication taken.
    - **Pollen alerts**: Inform patients about pollen levels in their area and offer advice on how to minimise exposure.
- Telemedicine   platforms:
    - **Virtual consultations**: Meet a specialist without travelling, which is essential for those living in remote areas.
    - **Remote   monitoring**: Allows doctors to monitor patients' vital signs and symptoms in real time.
- Medication   management applications:
    - **Medication   reminders**: Helps patients stick to their medication regime.

- **Drug information**: Informs patients about side effects, interactions and other important details.
- Platforms for therapeutic education:
  - **Videos and tutorials**: Training on self-injection, recognising the signs of anaphylaxis, etc.
  - **Education modules**: Learn more about allergies, immunology and prevention.
- Integration with electronic medical records:
  - **Data access**: Patients can consult their test results, prescriptions and medical history.
  - **Improved communication**: Facilitates communication between patients and healthcare professionals.

- Confidentiality and security:
  - **Data protection**: Understanding the security protocols in place to protect sensitive information.
  - **Informed consent**: Ensuring patients understand how their data is used.
- Future prospects and innovations:
  - **Artificial intelligence and machine learning**: how can these technologies be used to improve diagnosis and treatment?
  - **Augmented reality and virtual reality**: Potential use for training or to help patients understand their conditions.
- Advice on choosing the right application:
  - **Needs assessment**: Choosing an application tailored to the specific needs of the patient or professional.
  - **Criticism and recommendations**: Use the opinions of peers and users to assess the relevance of an application.

The use of apps and digital platforms in Allergology and Immunology has the potential to transform the way care is delivered. These tools offer not only convenience, but also an increased ability to personalise care, educate and engage patients in their own health. In an era of increasingly digitised medicine, staying at the forefront of these innovations is essential to delivering optimal care.

Telemedicine and remote care

Telemedicine has become an indispensable part of modern medicine, offering unprecedented flexibility and accessibility to medical care. In the field of Allergology and Immunology, it opens up new horizons for optimised care, transcending geographical and temporal barriers.

- Understanding telemedicine:
    - **Definition**: What is telemedicine and how does it differ from traditional care?
    - **History**: A brief overview of the evolution of telemedicine and its growing adoption.
- The benefits of telemedicine:
    - **Accessibility**: Breaking down geographical barriers, enabling patients in remote areas to access specialists.
    - **Efficiency**: Reduce waiting times, travel and optimise appointment management.
- Specific applications in Allergology and Immunology:
    - **Remote consultations**: discussion of symptoms, treatments and follow-up of allergic or immunocompromised patients.
    - **Therapeutic education**: Using digital platforms to educate patients about their condition, prevention and crisis management.

- Associated technologies:
    - **Videoconferencing platforms**: Tools for secure virtual consultations.
    - **Remote monitoring devices**: Monitors that allow vital signs or other relevant parameters to be monitored remotely.
- Challenges and concerns:
    - **Confidentiality and security**: guaranteeing the protection of sensitive medical information.
    - **Clinical limitations**: Recognising when a face-to-face consultation is necessary.
- Training and skills for nurses:
    - **Mastery of technological tools**: Acquire familiarity with the software and equipment used.
    - **Communication skills**: Communicating clearly and effectively via a screen.
- Integrating telemedicine into the care pathway:
    - **Coordination with traditional care**: How do virtual consultations fit into an overall care plan?
    - **Management of electronic medical records**: Ensuring a seamless transition of information between face-to-face and remote consultations.
- Future prospects:
    - **Technological innovations**: What are the next steps in telemedicine and how will they influence patient care?
    - **Acceptance and adoption**: The challenges and opportunities associated with the widespread use of telemedicine.

Telemedicine in Allergology and Immunology offers an incredible opportunity to deliver high quality care in a more accessible and flexible way. However, as with any technological advance, it must be approached with

163

caution, ensuring that clinical standards are maintained and that patient information is treated with the highest degree of confidentiality and security. By balancing these considerations, nurses can help shape a future where care is both personalised and universally accessible.

Technological innovations and their potential for the future

Allergology and immunology, like other medical disciplines, have undergone major technological advances in recent decades. These innovations have not only reshaped clinical practice, but have also broadened our understanding of the underlying mechanisms of allergic and immunological diseases.

- Technology at the service of diagnosis:
    - **Allergen detectors**: New portable devices for detecting allergens in the environment in real time.
    - **Molecular analysis**: Molecular tests offer a detailed understanding of the specific allergens involved, enabling a more accurate diagnosis.
- Advanced imaging:
    - **Functional magnetic resonance imaging (fMRI)**: Used to study brain reactions to allergens and to understand pain in autoimmune diseases.
    - **Positron emission tomography (PET)**: Useful for studying inflammation in various immunological diseases.

- Targeted and personalised therapies:
    - **Targeted immunotherapies**: Use of biotherapies, including monoclonal antibodies,

to specifically treat certain allergic and autoimmune diseases.

- **Gene therapy**: For hereditary immune deficiencies, offering the potential for curative treatment.
- Portable technology and patient monitoring:
  - **Home monitoring devices**: Portable monitors that allow patients to track their health, such as peak flow meters for asthma.
  - **Mobile applications**: For monitoring symptoms, managing medication and connecting with healthcare professionals.
- Artificial intelligence (AI) and big data:
  - **Predictive algorithms**: Using databases to predict allergic attacks or exacerbations of immunological diseases.
  - **Diagnostic aid**: AI systems that analyse symptoms and test results to aid diagnosis.
- Tele-allergology and digital platforms:
  - **Virtual consultations**: Using telemedicine to assess and manage patients.
  - **Patient education platforms**: Using virtual or augmented reality to educate about allergies and immunology.
- Biomaterials and drug delivery devices:
  - **Immunotherapy patches**: offering a less invasive alternative to injections.
  - Extended-release drug delivery systems: To ensure constant delivery of drugs.
- The future of innovation:
  - **Research and development**: Promising areas for innovation in Allergology and Immunology.
  - **Technology integration**: The challenges and opportunities associated with integrating new technologies into clinical practice.

With the rapid development of medical technologies, Allergology and Immunology are at the forefront of clinical advances. These innovations, while offering new methods of diagnosis and treatment, also require ongoing training for healthcare professionals to ensure optimal and safe use. The future promises more personalised, more precise and more preventive medicine for patients suffering from allergic and immunological conditions.

Chapter 19:
EDUCATIONAL ASPECTS
AND AWARENESS

Raising public awareness of allergies and immunological diseases

Raising public awareness of allergies and immunological diseases is essential to ensure the safety, well-being and general understanding of these often misunderstood conditions. Although the prevalence of allergies and immunological diseases is increasing worldwide, many myths and misunderstandings persist, making awareness all the more crucial.

- Why is awareness-raising important?
  - **Crisis prevention**: Understanding the signs and symptoms of allergic reactions can help prevent a serious crisis, such as anaphylaxis.
  - **Reducing stigma**: A better understanding of these conditions can help to reduce the stigma or lack of awareness associated with allergies and immunological diseases.
  - **Patient and family education**: Raising the awareness of those affected and those around them helps them to manage their condition more effectively.
- Awareness-raising methods:
  - **Media campaigns**: Use of advertising, press articles and reports to inform the public.
  - **Educational programmes in schools**: Incorporate allergy awareness into school curricula to educate from an early age.

- **Events and workshops**: Organise community forums, workshops and awareness-raising events.
- **World days**: Celebration of dedicated days, such as World Allergy Day, to highlight these conditions.
- Role of professional and non-governmental organisations:
    - These organisations can provide resources, guidelines and support for research, as well as running large-scale awareness campaigns.
- Working with influencers and celebrities:
    - Testimonials from influential people with allergies or immunological diseases can have a powerful impact on public perception.
- Development of online resources:
    - Creation of websites, applications and social media platforms offering reliable information and practical advice.
- Involvement of patients and their families:
    - Encourage patients and their families to share their experiences in order to humanise and personalise awareness-raising.
- Training for healthcare professionals:
    - Ensure that doctors, nurses and other healthcare professionals are well informed and equipped to educate their patients and the general public.

Raising awareness of these conditions requires a multifaceted approach, involving both high-level initiatives and community efforts. With increased awareness, we can hope for a better quality of life for those affected, a more empathetic response from society, and perhaps, in the long term, a reduction in prevalence through prevention and earlier intervention.

Patient and family education

Educating patients and their families is a fundamental pillar in the management of allergies and immunological diseases. By equipping people with the knowledge and tools they need to understand and manage their condition, we can increase their autonomy, improve their quality of life and reduce the risk of serious complications.

- The importance of education:
  - **Prevention**: Avoid allergenic exposure, be aware of the warning signs of a serious reaction.
  - **Effective self-management**: Educated patients are often more proactive in managing their condition.
  - **Stress reduction**: Understanding your illness reduces the anxiety associated with the unknown.
- Understanding the disease:
  - **Definition and causes**: What is an allergy or immunological disease? Why does it happen?
  - **Signs and symptoms**: Recognise typical symptoms for rapid intervention.
- Day-to-day management:
  - **Allergen avoidance**: Advice on eliminating common everyday allergens.
  - **Treatments**: How and when to take medicines, what to do if you forget, etc.
  - **Specific equipment**: For example, how to use an epinephrine auto-injector.
- Crisis action plan:
  - Establish a clear plan for allergic reactions, including the steps to follow and emergency numbers.

- Resources and support:
  - **Support groups**: To share experiences and advice.
  - **Digital applications and tools**: For monitoring symptoms, recognising allergens, etc.
  - **Literature**: Books, brochures, reliable websites to learn more.
- Family education:
  - **First aid training**: In the event of a serious allergic reaction, every second counts.
  - **Tips for everyday life**: Cooking for an allergic family member, recognising the signs of a reaction, etc.
  - **Emotional management**: Supporting the patient, managing anxiety or stress associated with the condition.
- Working with healthcare professionals:
  - **Regular consultations**: to ensure medical follow-up and discuss any concerns.
  - **Keeping up to date**: Recommendations and treatments evolve with research; it's essential to stay informed.
- Involvement in the community:
  - **Raising awareness**: Educating the wider community can help create a safer environment for those suffering from allergies or immunological diseases.

Educating patients and their families is an ongoing process. As patients grow, as their condition evolves or as new scientific discoveries emerge, their educational needs change. The approach must therefore be flexible, personalised and always focused on the patient's well-being and safety.

Continuing education programmes for nurses

In the dynamic and ever-changing world of medicine, continuing education is essential to ensure that nurses maintain and improve their expertise, keep up to date with the latest medical advances and ensure optimal patient care. Continuing education programmes for Allergology and Immunology nurses focus on a range of topics from updating clinical skills to understanding the latest research.

- The importance of ongoing training:
  - **Quality of care**: Maintaining a high level of competence to ensure the best possible care for patients.
  - **Keeping up to date**: Science and medicine evolve rapidly, so keeping up to date is essential.
  - **Career development**: Opportunities to advance your career or specialise further.
- Clinical modules:
  - **Advanced techniques**: For example, the administration of innovative biological treatments or immunotherapies.
  - **Emergency management**: In-depth training on emergency situations specific to Allergology and Immunology, such as severe anaphylaxis.
- Research updates:
  - **Latest discoveries**: How do new discoveries influence clinical practice?
  - **Case studies**: Detailed analysis of case studies to understand the nuances of patient management.

- Non-clinical skills:
  - **Communication**: Improving communication skills for better interaction with patients, families and the medical team.
  - **Stress management**: Techniques for managing stress and avoiding burn-out in a demanding medical environment.
- Emerging technologies:
  - **Training on new equipment**: For example, the use of innovative medical devices or patient monitoring software.
  - **Telemedicine**: How do you provide remote care while maintaining quality?
- Interdisciplinary collaboration:
  - **Working with other specialties**: Understanding the roles and responsibilities of other medical specialties and how to collaborate effectively.
  - **Joint seminars**: Training courses combining different specialities for a more holistic approach to care.
- Ethics training:
  - **Specific ethical considerations**: For example, management of patient information, informed consent for experimental treatments.
- Specialised modules:
  - **Paediatric Allergology and Immunology**: Focusing on the particularities of caring for children.
  - **Uncommon allergies: A** deeper understanding of less common but just as crucial allergies.
- Participation in conferences and workshops:
  - **Networking**: Meet other professionals in the field to exchange experience and knowledge.
  - **Practical workshops**: interactive, hands-on learning.

Continuing education is a responsibility and a privilege for nurses. Not only does it guarantee optimal patient care, it also provides nurses with opportunities for professional and personal development, reinforcing their essential role within the medical team.

The importance of popularising science

In a world saturated with information, where every individual has access to a multitude of sources via the Internet, television, social networks, etc., it is crucial to be able to distinguish real facts from myths or erroneous information. Popular science plays a key role here. But what is popular science, and why is it so essential?

- **Definition of popular science:**
  - Science popularisation is the art of making scientific information accessible to a non-specialist audience. It transforms technical jargon and complex concepts into simple, understandable terms, without distorting scientific reality.
- **Breaking down the barrier between science and the public:**
  - Many people perceive science as elitist or out of reach. Popularising science makes it accessible, demystifying concepts that can seem intimidating.
- **Promoting education:**
  - Making science attractive and accessible encourages curiosity and lifelong learning. Young people, in particular, can be inspired to pursue careers in science or technology.
- **Combating misinformation:**
  - With the proliferation of "fake news", it is essential to have reliable and understandable

sources that clearly demonstrate the facts. Science popularisers are often at the forefront of countering myths and misinformation.

- **Informed decision-making:**
  - Whether it's understanding the implications of climate change, deciding whether to get vaccinated or supporting stem cell research, an informed population is better equipped to make informed decisions on issues that affect their daily lives.
- **Encouraging dialogue:**
  - By establishing a common ground on which scientists and non-scientists can interact, popularisation encourages dialogue. It enables fruitful exchanges, encouraging questions, mutual understanding and collaboration.
- **Promoting research:**
  - Sharing scientific discoveries with the general public enhances the value of researchers' work. This can lead to increased support for science, both in terms of funding and general appreciation.
- **Ethical reflection:**
  - Popularisation also makes it possible to raise ethical issues and encourage the general public to think about the implications of scientific research and discoveries.
- **Developments in general culture:**
  - A society that understands and appreciates science is a society that values knowledge, innovation and critical thinking.

Science popularisation is a bridge between the complex world of research and the general public. It enlightens, inspires and engages, helping to create an informed, inquisitive and forward-looking society. In a world where science is playing an increasingly central role, the ability to communicate effectively on these subjects is becoming not just valuable, but essential.

Chapter 20:
ALLERGOLOGY EMERGENCIES AND IMMUNOLOGY

Recognising an anaphylactic reaction

Anaphylaxis is a serious and potentially fatal allergic reaction that develops rapidly after exposure to an allergen. It affects several organs simultaneously and requires immediate medical intervention. Early recognition of the signs and symptoms of anaphylaxis can save lives. Here's how to recognise it.

- Skin symptoms:
    - Sudden redness or paleness of the skin
    - Hives or rash
    - Itching, particularly of the palms or soles
- Respiratory symptoms:
    - Difficulty breathing or shortness of breath
    - Wheezing or noise when breathing
    - Persistent cough
    - Sensation of constriction or tightness in the throat
    - Hoarse voice
- Cardiovascular symptoms:
    - Rapid or irregular pulse
    - Chest pain or tightness
    - Dizziness, weakness or fainting
    - Fall in blood pressure
- Digestive symptoms:
    - Nausea or vomiting
    - Diarrhoea
    - Abdominal pain
- Neurological symptoms:
    - Headaches

- A feeling of impending doom, a strange sensation of apprehension or fear
- Confusion or altered consciousness
- Other signs:
  - Swollen eyes or face
  - Winding
  - Difficulty swallowing

When you recognise these symptoms, it's essential to act quickly:

- **Call the emergency services**: If you suspect anaphylaxis, call the emergency services immediately.
- **Administering an epinephrine auto-injector**: If the sufferer has an epinephrine auto-injector (such as an EpiPen), it should be used without delay. Follow the instructions supplied with the auto-injector.
- **Put the person in a safe position**: Lay the person down with their legs raised, unless they are having difficulty breathing or are vomiting. In this case, it is preferable to put the person in a sitting position to facilitate breathing.
- **Stay with the person**: Never leave a person showing signs of anaphylaxis alone.
- Avoid giving water or food: This could aggravate the symptoms.

Prevention is the most effective way of managing the risk of anaphylaxis. It is essential to know your allergens, avoid exposure and always have an epinephrine auto-injector to hand if you are at risk.

Emergency protocols for anaphylactic shock

Anaphylactic shock is the most serious form of anaphylactic reaction, manifesting as acute circulatory failure and potentially leading to cardiac arrest. Prompt and appropriate treatment is vital. Here is a typical emergency protocol for anaphylactic shock:

- Shock recognition:
    - Sudden onset of symptoms
    - Symptoms affecting several organ systems (skin, respiratory, cardiovascular, digestive, etc.)
    - Serious symptoms such as difficulty breathing, confusion, paleness or cyanosis, weakness or collapse
- Call emergency services immediately:
    - Seek help, call the emergency services and inform them that anaphylactic shock is suspected.
- Position the patient:
    - If the person is breathing normally and is not in respiratory distress, lay them down with their legs elevated.
    - If the person has difficulty breathing or is vomiting, put them in a semi-seated position to make breathing easier.
- Epinephrine   auto-injector:
    - If the patient has an epinephrine auto-injector (EpiPen, Jext, Anapen, etc.), administer it immediately, following the manufacturer's instructions.
    - Make sure you note the time of injection.
- Clear the airways:
    - If the patient is conscious but in respiratory distress, ask them to take deep breaths.
    - If the person is not breathing or is breathing irregularly, start cardiopulmonary resuscitation (CPR).
- **Avoid administering other medicines** without clear medical instructions, unless they are part of the patient's allergy action plan.
- Monitor the patient:

- Stay with the patient until help arrives.
- Be prepared to administer a second dose of epinephrine after 5 to 15 minutes if symptoms do not improve or worsen.
- Information for emergency services:
  - When the emergency services arrive, inform them of the medication administered, the time of administration and the progression of symptoms.
- Medical transport:
  - Even if symptoms improve after the administration of epinephrine, the person should be taken to hospital for further observation, as symptoms may reappear.
- Future prevention:
- Once the patient is stabilised, it is crucial to address future prevention, recognition of triggers, ownership and correct use of an epinephrine auto-injector, and the need for a well-defined allergy action plan.

Every minute counts in the event of anaphylactic shock. Rapid intervention, following a well-defined protocol, can save lives.

Managing serious complications following immunotherapy

Immunotherapy, often referred to as desensitisation, has transformed the treatment of many allergic diseases. However, as with any medical treatment, immunotherapy is not without risks. Serious complications, although rare, can occur. Here are some of them, along with recommendations for their management:

- Anaphylactic reactions :
  - The most feared reaction is anaphylaxis. It requires immediate treatment with epinephrine, a call to the emergency room and monitoring of the patient.
  - If such a reaction occurs, the continuation of immunotherapy must be reconsidered and discussed with the patient.
- Systemic reactions :
  - These may include symptoms such as generalised skin rashes, breathing difficulties, abdominal pain, etc.
  - Treatment varies according to the severity of symptoms, but may include antihistamines, corticosteroids and, in the most severe cases, epinephrine.
- Local reactions :
  - These reactions are generally less severe, but may be painful or uncomfortable. They may include redness, swelling or itching at the injection site.
  - Local or oral antihistamines can help relieve these symptoms.
- Cytokine release syndrome :
  - Although more common with certain forms of cancer immunotherapy, this syndrome can lead to fever, fatigue, muscle aches and other flu-like symptoms.
  - It is generally treated with medication to reduce fever and pain, and with appropriate hydration.
- Complication management :
  - Rapid assessment and management are essential.
  - All patients receiving immunotherapy must be informed of the signs and symptoms of serious complications and know when and how to seek medical help.

- It is crucial that staff administering immunotherapy are trained to recognise and manage complications.
- Reassessment of treatment :
  - If complications arise, immunotherapy should be reassessed. This could include dose adjustments, extension of the post-injection observation period or, in some cases, discontinuation of immunotherapy.
- Prevention of complications :
  - A thorough assessment of the patient before starting immunotherapy, together with regular monitoring, can help reduce the risk of complications.
  - Administering gradually increasing doses and following established protocols also helps to minimise risks.

The key to managing serious complications following immunotherapy is preparation. Having a plan in place, being aware of the risks and being ready to intervene quickly can make the difference between a controlled complication and a potentially fatal situation.

Handling emergencies in and out of hospital

The management of a medical emergency can vary depending on whether it occurs in or out of hospital. Both contexts present unique challenges and advantages, and responsiveness and preparedness are essential in both cases.

In hospitals:
- Availability of resources :
    - The major advantage of a hospital emergency is the rapid availability of medical resources, equipment and trained staff.
- Quick response:
    - In most hospitals, a rapid response team or resuscitation team is in place to respond immediately to emergencies.
- Access to medical records :
    - Electronic medical records can quickly provide vital information on a patient's medical history, allergies, medication, etc.
- Internal transfer :
    - If necessary, patients can be rapidly transferred to intensive care units or other specialist departments.

Outside hospitals:
- First speakers:
    - First responders, such as paramedics, play a crucial role in stabilising the patient and providing first aid.
- Communication :
    - Coordination with emergency call centres (such as 112 in Europe or 911 in North America) is vital. They provide real-time instructions and alert the appropriate emergency services.
- Transport challenges :
    - Fast and safe transport to the nearest hospital is essential. This can be complicated by distance, traffic, weather conditions, etc.
- Resource limitations :
    - Ambulances are well equipped, but they do not have all the resources of a hospital. The aim is often to stabilise the patient for transport.

- First aid training :
  - Bystanders to an emergency can play a crucial role if they are trained in first aid. Basic manoeuvres such as cardiopulmonary resuscitation (CPR) or the use of an automated external defibrillator (AED) can save lives while waiting for help to arrive.

Advice on effective care:
- **Training**: Healthcare professionals and the general public should consider first aid and CPR training.
- **Preparation**: Hospitals must regularly carry out emergency simulations to ensure that staff know how to react.
- **Communication**: Clear and effective communication between all stakeholders is essential.
- **Updating skills**: Emergency protocols evolve with time and research. Ongoing training is therefore essential.

Dealing with emergencies, whether in or out of hospital, requires effective responsiveness, preparation and coordination to ensure the best possible outcome for the patient.

Chapter 21:
FOOD ALLERGIES

Main food allergens
and their recognition

Food allergies are immune reactions to certain proteins in food. These reactions can range from simple skin irritation to potentially fatal symptoms such as anaphylactic shock. Recognising these allergens is crucial to preventing and managing allergic reactions.

The main food allergens:
- Eggs :
  - Particularly the proteins contained in egg whites. Reactions often vary in severity.
- Milk :
  - Some people are allergic to casein or other proteins present in cow's milk. This is not to be confused with lactose intolerance, which is an inability to digest milk sugar.
- Peanuts :
  - These are among the most common and often the most serious allergies, which can lead to anaphylactic shock.
- Nuts :
  - Such as cashews, hazelnuts, almonds and pecans. Reactions can be severe.
- Soya :
  - Soya proteins can cause reactions in some people, especially children, although many children outgrow them during childhood.

- Wheat :
  - Wheat allergy is different from coeliac disease. It is triggered by wheat proteins and not by gluten.
- Fish :
  - Especially in adults, and reactions are often severe.
- Crustaceans :
  - Like prawns, crabs and lobsters. This allergy is more common in adults than in children.

Recognition of food allergens:
- Reading labels :
  - Always check food labels to identify potential allergens. In many countries, it is compulsory to indicate the presence of the main allergens on the packaging.
- Ask questions during meals out:
  - If you eat in a restaurant or at someone's home, always ask how the food is prepared and what ingredients are used.
- Avoid cross-contamination:
  - Be sure to clean all utensils and cooking surfaces thoroughly after use for potential allergens.
- Allergy tests :
  - Skin tests or blood tests can help identify food allergens. Consult an allergist for a precise diagnosis.
- Keep a food diary:
  - If you suspect a food allergy, keep a diary of what you eat and note any symptoms you may experience. This can help isolate the potential allergen.

Recognising and avoiding allergens is the key to preventing allergic reactions. When in doubt, it's always best to consult a specialist for appropriate advice and support.

The importance of a food history

A dietary history is an essential medical procedure which aims to collect and evaluate information about an individual's food consumption in a systematic and detailed way. It provides a precise picture of eating habits, preferences, aversions and any reactions or symptoms associated with the consumption of certain foods. Here's why it's so important:

1. Diagnosis of food allergies and intolerances :
A food history is the first crucial step in diagnosing allergies and intolerances. By listening carefully to the patient describe their symptoms after eating certain foods, the practitioner can identify trends or potential triggers.

2. Disease prevention :
Studies have shown that diet plays a significant role in the prevention of many diseases, such as cardiovascular disease, diabetes and certain types of cancer. A dietary history can help identify risks and guide patients towards healthier food choices.

3. Weight management :
Obesity is a major public health concern. By understanding a patient's eating habits, healthcare professionals can recommend dietary changes that promote **weight** loss **or the maintenance of a healthy weight.**

4. Optimising nutrition :
For patients with specific nutritional needs, such as pregnant women, athletes or the elderly, a detailed dietary history enables dietary recommendations to be tailored to their needs.

5. Monitoring malnutrition :
In certain vulnerable populations, such as the elderly, children or people suffering from chronic illnesses, a dietary history is a valuable tool for detecting signs of malnutrition or nutritional deficiencies.

6. Adapting medical treatments :
Some medicines can interact with foods or nutrients. An accurate dietary history enables treatments to be adjusted accordingly.

7. Evaluating eating habits :
In addition to the simple consumption of food, the history may reveal eating disorders such as bulimia or anorexia, which require specific treatment.

8. Establishing a relationship of trust :
The dietary history is a time for exchange between the patient and the healthcare professional. It allows a relationship of trust to be established, which is essential to the success of any dietetic or medical intervention.

A dietary history is an essential tool for understanding a patient's state of health, habits and needs. It enables individualised, tailored care to be provided, guaranteeing better quality of care. It is crucial for healthcare professionals to devote the necessary time and attention to it.

Interventions
in the event of an allergic reaction to food

When faced with a food-allergic reaction, it is crucial to act quickly and effectively to prevent symptoms from worsening and to save lives in the event of a severe reaction. Here is a list of actions to take:

1. Assessment of severity :
  • Identify the symptoms. Food allergic reactions can manifest themselves as itching, redness, swelling (face, lips, tongue), breathing difficulties, vomiting, diarrhoea, malaise, palpitations, a drop in blood pressure, and so on.

2. Stop eating the allergen :
   - If the person continues to eat the food responsible, it is essential to ask them to stop immediately.
3. Administer an antihistamine :
   - If symptoms are mild (skin rash, itching), an oral antihistamine may be administered, provided it has been prescribed in advance by a doctor.
4. Using the epinephrine auto-injector :
   - In the event of severe symptoms or anaphylaxis (severe and rapid allergic reaction), if the person has an epinephrine auto-injector (such as the EpiPen), it should be used immediately according to the instructions provided by the doctor.
5. Call emergency services :
   - Call your local emergency number (such as 112 in Europe or 911 in the United States) at the first sign of a severe reaction. Do not attempt to transport the person to hospital yourself.
6. Put the person in a safe position:
   - If the person is conscious, put them in a comfortable position, prevent them from drinking or eating anything, and try to reassure them.
   - If she loses consciousness, put her in the lateral position.
7. Continuous monitoring :
   - Keep an eye on the person's condition until help arrives. Symptoms may worsen or return even after an apparent improvement.
8. Inform emergency services :
   - When the emergency services arrive, inform them of the food consumed, the time taken for symptoms to appear, the medication administered (including the dose of epinephrine, if used) and any other relevant details.
9. Medical consultation :
   - Even after the reaction has stabilised, the patient should consult a doctor or allergist to discuss the reaction and adjust the treatment plan if necessary.

It is crucial that anyone with a food allergy, and those around them, are properly trained to recognise symptoms and know how to react in the event of a crisis. Proper training can mean the difference between life and death in the event of a severe allergic reaction.

Patient and family education to prevent exposure

Educating patients and their families is a fundamental part of preventing allergenic exposure. Here are some key steps and tips to ensure effective education:

1. Understanding allergies :
   * Start by clearly explaining what an allergy is, how the immune system reacts to an allergen and why certain reactions can be serious.
2. Identification of the allergen :
   * Once an allergy has been diagnosed, it is essential to teach the patient and his or her family how to recognise the allergen, whether it is a food, medicine, chemical or other product.
3. Reading the labels :
   * For food allergies, teach how to read and interpret product labels correctly. Focus on checking for hidden ingredients or traces of allergens.
4. Home management :
   * Provide advice on how to minimise exposure to the allergen at home. This could include recommendations on cleaning, food storage or avoiding certain products.
5. Allergy action plan :
   * Draw up a personalised action plan for each patient, detailing the steps to be taken in the event of exposure to the allergen. This plan should be accessible and understandable to all family members.

6. Training in the use of medicines :
   - If the patient has emergency medication, such as an epinephrine auto-injector, make sure they and their family know how and when to use it.
7. School and social education :
   - Make families aware of the importance of communicating with schools, clubs, friends and other institutions about allergies. Provide them with explanatory documents or letters if necessary.
8. Managing social situations :
   - Give advice on how to manage outings, restaurant meals or trips. This may include recommendations on communicating with staff or preparing safe meals in advance.
9. Know the signs and symptoms :
   - Make sure that patients and their families recognise the early signs of an allergic reaction and know when and how to seek help.
10. Encouraging responsibility :
    - Encourage patients, especially younger ones, to take their allergy seriously and be proactive in managing their health.
11. Resources and support :
    - Refer patients and families to support groups, educational websites or other resources that can help them better manage and understand allergy.

Education is a powerful weapon in the prevention of allergenic exposure. By providing the necessary tools and knowledge, you enable patients and their families to live safely and independently while effectively managing their allergies.

Chapter 22:
PAEDIATRIC ALLERGOLOGY AND IMMUNOLOGY

Special features paediatric care

The care of children with allergies or immunological problems differs from that of adults in several respects. Here are the particularities of this specific population:

1. Clinical presentation :
   * The symptoms of allergies or immune disorders in children may differ from those in adults. For example, atopic dermatitis or eczema is common in young children, while allergic asthma is more common in older children.
2. Diagnosis :
   * Allergological and immunological tests must be adapted to the child's age. What's more, children may not be able to express their symptoms clearly, so careful observation is essential.
3. Drug administration :
   * Drug dosages for children are generally based on their weight, requiring special attention to ensure accurate administration.
4. Development of the immune system :
   * Children's immune systems are still developing, which can affect how they react to allergens and how their allergies develop over time.
5. Development of allergies :
   * Some allergies can dissipate over time. For example, many children outgrow an allergy to milk or eggs as they grow up.

6. Education :
   - Educating children about their condition requires a different approach to adults. It's about making information accessible while encouraging them to take age-appropriate responsibility.
7. Families involved :
   - The involvement of parents or guardians is essential in the management of allergies and immune disorders in children. They play a central role in monitoring, administering medication and preventing exposure.
8. School environment :
   - It is crucial to communicate with teachers, school officials and other parents to ensure that the school environment is safe for the child.
9. Psychosocial aspects :
   - Children with allergies or immune disorders may feel isolated or different from their peers. Psychological and social support may be needed to help the child manage these feelings.
10. Diet :
   - If the child has food allergies, this may require special attention in terms of nutrition to ensure that he or she receives all the essential nutrients while avoiding allergens.
11. Emergency plans :
   - Given that children spend a lot of time at school or in other activities, it is vital to have a clearly defined emergency action plan that is communicated to everyone involved.
12. Ethical aspects :
   - As with any medical intervention in children, it is essential to take ethical issues into account, particularly with regard to consent and assent.

Paediatric allergology and immunology care requires a holistic approach that takes into account the unique needs of the child and his or her family. The main aim is to ensure the child's safety and well-being, while offering the best possible quality of life.

Allergies in infants and young children

In infants and young children, the immune system is still developing. This can make them more vulnerable to certain allergies, even though some of them may disappear over time. Here's an overview of common allergies in this age group, along with advice on how to manage them.

1. Food allergies :
   - **Symptoms**: Eczema, urticaria, vomiting, diarrhoea, angioedema and, in extreme cases, anaphylactic shock.
   - **Common allergens** : Cow's milk, eggs, nuts, peanuts, fish, soya, wheat.
   - **Management**: Eliminating the allergen from the diet, educating parents about reading labels, wearing an allergy alert bracelet.
2. Atopic dermatitis (eczema) :
   - **Symptoms**: Dry, red and itchy skin. Can become infected if scratched.
   - **Management**: Moisturising the skin, topical creams, avoiding triggers such as certain soaps or fabrics.
3. Allergy to house dust mites :
   - **Symptoms**: Sneezing, runny nose, itchy eyes.
   - **Management**: Use dust mite-proof covers for bedding, vacuum frequently, avoid lint.
4. Allergic rhinitis :
   - **Symptoms**: Sneezing, nasal congestion, watery eyes.
   - **Management**: Identification and avoidance of allergens, use of antihistamines with the advice of the paediatrician.

5. Asthma :
- Although asthma is not an allergy, it is often linked to allergies.
- **Symptoms**: Coughing, wheezing, shortness of breath.
- **Management**: Use of inhalers, identification and avoidance of triggers.

Advice for parents:
- **Consultation**: If you suspect your child has an allergy, consult an allergist or paediatrician for tests and advice.
- **Breast-feeding**: Exclusive breast-feeding for at least the first 6 months can help prevent certain allergies.
- **Introducing allergens**: Follow your paediatrician's recommendations for introducing potential allergens into your child's diet.
- **Avoid allergens**: Learn to recognise and avoid common allergens in food and the environment.
- **Action plan**: Draw up an allergy action plan, especially if your child has severe reactions. Make sure your child's carers are aware of this plan.

Allergies in infants and young children can be worrying for parents. However, with early identification, appropriate management and education, many children can live normal, happy lives while managing their allergies. In some cases, children can even outgrow their allergies over time.

Psychological support for children and their families

When a child is diagnosed with an allergy, it affects not just the child, but the whole family. The psychological impact can be significant. Understanding and managing these emotional aspects is crucial to the well-being of the child and his or her family.

1. Impact on the child:
   - **Fear and anxiety**: Fear of an allergic reaction can cause anxiety in children, especially at social events such as birthdays.
   - **Social isolation**: Children may feel different from their peers and choose to isolate themselves to avoid exposure to allergens.
   - **Feeling stigmatised**: The child may feel stigmatised or ashamed because of their condition.
2. Impact on the family:
   - **Parental stress**: Parents may feel constant anxiety about their child's health, especially when he or she is not at home.
   - **Siblings**: Siblings may feel neglected or jealous of the extra attention given to the allergic child. They may also feel afraid for their brother or sister.
   - **Daily pressures**: Preparing meals, reading labels, organising outings... It can all be exhausting for parents.
3. Psychological support:
   - **Individual therapy**: A psychologist can help children manage their fears and boost their self-confidence.
   - **Family therapy**: This helps to deal with family tensions and strengthen support within the family.
   - **Support groups**: Sharing experiences with other families facing the same challenges can be beneficial.
4. Strategies for parents:
   - **Open communication**: Encourage your child to express fears and concerns.
   - **Education**: Educate children about their condition so that they can protect themselves.
   - **Inclusion**: Make sure the child participates in as many activities as possible. Work with schools and clubs to ensure a safe environment.
   - **Positive reinforcement**: Praise your child when he manages his condition well.

5. Peer education:
  - Making classmates and teachers aware of the child's condition can help to create a more understanding environment.
6. Resources:
  - Look for associations and organisations that offer support, workshops and resources for allergic children and their families.

Managing a child's allergy requires a holistic approach that encompasses not only medical treatment, but also emotional and psychological support. By empowering children and their families with the right tools and support, they can successfully navigate the challenges presented by allergies and lead fulfilling lives.

Transition to adult care

The transition from paediatric to adult care is a delicate and crucial stage in the life of a patient suffering from allergic or immunological disorders. It marks the transition from a generally more protective environment to one where autonomy and individual responsibility are given greater prominence. This transition must be approached with care to ensure continuity of care and preserve the patient's quality of life.

1. Preparing for the transition:
  - **Early education**: From adolescence onwards, patients should be informed of the need for transition and what it entails. They should be helped to understand their condition, their treatments and the responsibilities that go with them.
  - **Planning**: A transition plan should be drawn up well before the age of majority. This plan should include an

assessment of the patient's skills, needs and concerns.

2. Role of healthcare professionals:
   - **Coordination**: Healthcare professionals, whether in paediatrics or adult medicine, should work together to ensure a smooth transition.
   - **Close follow-up**: At the beginning of the transition, more frequent appointments may be necessary to ensure that the patient is adapting well to the new care environment.

3. Patient autonomy:
   - **Medication management**: Patients should be trained to manage their own medication, recognise symptoms and know when and how to seek help.
   - **Empowerment**: Encouraging patients to take responsibility for their medical appointments, prescription renewals and interactions with the healthcare system.

4. Emotional support:
   - **Worry and anxiety**: The transition to adult care can be worrying. Offering psychological support can help address these feelings.
   - **Support groups**: Joining a support group for young adults facing similar challenges can be beneficial.

5. Challenges specific to the transition:
   - **Institutional changes**: Moving from a children's hospital to an adult hospital can be intimidating. A preliminary visit can help to allay certain fears.
   - **Confidentiality**: Adults have greater rights to confidentiality, which may require adjustments, particularly for parents who are used to being closely involved.

6. The role of parents and carers:
   - **Letting go gradually**: Encouraging independence does not mean abandoning support. Parents need to strike a balance between encouraging independence and offering the necessary help.

The transition from paediatric to adult care is a major step. Careful preparation, open communication and constant support can help ensure that this transition goes as smoothly as possible, putting patients on the road to managing their health independently and effectively in adulthood.

Chapter 23:
PRIMARY IMMUNODEFICIENCIES

Recognition of the main immunodeficiency syndromes

Immunodeficiency syndromes refer to a group of diseases in which the immune system does not function properly or is insufficient, exposing the individual to recurrent and sometimes serious infections. These deficiencies may be innate (present from birth) or acquired. Early recognition of these syndromes is essential if appropriate treatment is to be put in place and complications prevented.

1. Primary immune deficiency (PID):
DIPs are generally genetic in origin and often appear in childhood.
- Antibody deficiency:
    - *X-linked globulinaemia (Bruton)*: absence of immunoglobulins in the blood.
    - *Variable common deficiency*: reduction in several types of immunoglobulin.
- Combined losses:
    - *DiGeorge syndrome:* absence or hypoplasia of the thymus leading to T-cell deficiency.
    - Severe combined immunodeficiency (SCID): deficiency of both B and T cells.
- Phagocytic deficiencies:
    - *Chronic granulomatous disease*: inability of neutrophils to destroy certain bacteria or fungi.
- Immune activation and auto-inflammatory syndromes:
    - *Hyper IgM syndrome*: increase in IgM and decrease in other immunoglobulins.

2. Secondary (or acquired) immune deficiencies:
Unlike DIPs, secondary immune deficiencies result from an external cause.

- **HIV/AIDS**: the human immunodeficiency virus attacks and destroys CD4 cells, which are essential for the immune response.
- **Immunosuppressive treatments**: drugs such as corticosteroids, post-transplant immunosuppressants or certain anti-cancer agents can affect the immune system.
- **Cancers**: some cancers, particularly leukaemia and lymphoma, can weaken the immune response.
- **Malnutrition**: inadequate nutritional intake can compromise immune function.
- **Chronic infections**: certain infections, such as tuberculosis, can weaken the immune system over time.

Evocative signs:
- Recurrent or unusually serious infections.
- Infections caused by opportunistic pathogens.
- Delayed growth or development in children.
- Autoimmune manifestations.
- Granulomas in various organs.

When faced with repeated, unusual or severe infections, it is essential to suspect immunodeficiency. A full immune assessment is often necessary to confirm the diagnosis. Early management can considerably improve patients' quality of life and reduce the risk of serious complications.

Patient follow-up
with immunodeficiency

Regular monitoring of patients suffering from immunodeficiency is crucial to assess the progress of the disease, prevent complications, adjust treatment and ensure the patient's general well-being. The complexity of this care requires a multidisciplinary approach.

1. Regular clinical assessment :
   - **Frequency of consultations** : Patients may require frequent consultations, depending on the severity of their condition and the type of immunodeficiency.
   - **Infection monitoring**: It is essential to detect any infection early so that it can be treated before it gets worse.
   - **Development assessment** : Regular monitoring of children's physical and mental development is crucial.
2. Biological monitoring :
   - **Immunological tests**: to assess the functioning and condition of the immune system.
   - **Haemogram**: To monitor the levels of different blood cells.
   - **Serology**: To detect certain infections.
3. Infection prevention :
   - **Vaccinations**: Appropriate vaccinations may be necessary, particularly to avoid certain infections.
   - **Antimicrobial prophylaxis**: Some patients may require long-term prophylaxis to prevent specific infections.
   - **Hygiene measures**: Advice on the hygiene measures to adopt to minimise the risk of infection.
4. Specific treatments :
   - **Substitutive therapy**: such as intravenous or subcutaneous immunoglobulins for patients with an antibody deficiency.
   - **Immunomodulating treatments**: To adjust the activity of the immune system.
   - **Transplantation**: such as bone marrow transplants for severe combined immunodeficiency.
5. Psychosocial follow-up :
   - **Psychological support**: Many patients and their families need psychological support to help them

cope with their diagnosis and the challenges of everyday life.
- **Adapting to school or work**: Children may need special arrangements at school.

6. Coordination with other specialists :
- Given that immunodeficiency can affect various organs and systems, close coordination with other specialists (pulmonologists, gastroenterologists, dermatologists, etc.) is often necessary.

7. Patient and family education :
- It is essential to educate the patient and his or her family about the disease, the warning signs of possible infection, the management of medication and the measures to be taken to minimise risks.

Monitoring patients with immunodeficiency is a complex process that requires a personalised approach. Collaboration between healthcare professionals, patients and their families is the key to ensuring the best possible quality of life for these patients.

Infection prevention in these patients

Patients with immunodeficiency are particularly vulnerable to infection because of the reduced or absent capacity of their immune system to fight pathogens. Infection prevention is therefore a key element in their management. Here are some essential measures for preventing infections in these patients:

1. Appropriate vaccinations :
- Ensure that the patient receives all the recommended vaccines, while avoiding live attenuated vaccines

which could be dangerous for certain immunocompromised patients.

- Monitor responses to vaccines to ensure they are effective.

2. Antimicrobial prophylaxis :
   - Administer antimicrobial drugs as a preventive measure to avoid specific infections, particularly in high-risk patients.

3. Strict hygiene measures :
   - Practice good hand hygiene using soap and water or alcohol-based hand sanitisers.
   - Avoid touching the face, especially the eyes, nose and mouth.
   - Keep wounds clean and well covered.

4. Protection against respiratory infections :
   - Avoid crowds and public places during flu seasons or epidemics.
   - Wear a mask when visiting hospitals or other high-risk environments.
   - Encourage family members and friends to get vaccinated against flu to create a barrier of protection.

5. Secure power supply :
   - Favour cooked or well-washed foods.
   - Avoid high-risk foods such as raw meat, raw fish, raw eggs and unpasteurised dairy products.

6. Drinking water :
   - Make sure you only drink purified or boiled water, especially in areas where drinking water may be contaminated.

7. Prevention of skin infections :
   - Avoid prolonged bathing and standing water.
   - Use moisturising lotions to prevent chapping and cracking of the skin.
   - Watch out for signs of infection such as redness, heat, swelling or pain.

8. Prevention of opportunistic infections :
   - Certain pathogens, generally harmless to a healthy person, can cause serious illness in

immunocompromised patients. Their identification and preventive treatment can be essential.

9. Education and awareness :
- Educate patients and their families about the risks of infection and the preventive measures to adopt.
- Encourage patients to recognise the first signs of infection so that they can be treated quickly.

10. Coordination with other specialists :
- Working closely with other health professionals to ensure comprehensive care and prevent infections.

Preventing infections in immunodeficient patients requires a proactive, individualised and multidisciplinary approach to ensure their safety and well-being.

Patient education and support and their families

Educating patients and their families is essential in the management of allergies and immunological diseases. It aims not only to inform, but also to empower patients, making them active players in their own health. Here are some key elements of this education, together with strategies for providing appropriate support:

1. Information on the illness or allergy :
- Provide a clear and understandable explanation of the disease, its symptoms and its course.
- Explain potential triggers or specific allergens linked to the condition.

2. Medication management :
- Teaching the correct use of medicines, their dosage, frequency and possible side effects.
- In the case of allergies, show how to use an epinephrine auto-injector, if prescribed.

3. Recognising warning signs :
   - Educate patients and their families on how to identify the early signs of a severe allergic reaction or exacerbation of the disease, and when to seek medical help.
4. Prevention strategies :
   - Give advice on avoiding allergens, proper nutrition and other preventive measures.
5. Managing fear and anxiety :
   - Offering psychological support to help patients and families deal with the uncertainty, fear and anxiety associated with the disease.
6. Encouraging autonomy :
   - Educate patients, particularly children and adolescents, to gradually take charge of their own health, including recognising symptoms and managing medication.
7. Support groups :
   - Referring patients and their families to local or national support groups, where they can talk to other people in similar situations.
8. Educational resources :
   - Provide brochures, videos, websites and other educational resources to further their knowledge.
9. Personalised action plan :
   - Draw up an action plan with the patient in the event of a crisis or exacerbation, and ensure that it is clearly understood and accessible to family and friends.
10. Promoting open dialogue :
    - Encourage patients and their families to ask questions, share concerns and establish regular communication with healthcare professionals.

Educating patients and their families is a fundamental part of allergology and immunology care. It not only helps to improve patients' quality of life, but also to prevent potentially serious complications. An empathetic, patient and caring approach is essential to establish a relationship of trust, which will be beneficial to the overall management of the patient.

Chapter 24:
QUALITY OF LIFE
AND LONG-TERM MONITORING

Assessing the quality of life of allergic and immunocompromised patients

Quality of life is an essential indicator of overall patient care. For those who suffer from allergies or are immunocompromised, their medical condition can have a major impact on their physical, emotional, social and functional well-being. Assessing their quality of life goes far beyond simply measuring symptoms. Here's how this assessment can be approached:

1. Standardised questionnaires :
There are specific questionnaires for assessing the quality of life of allergic or immunocompromised patients. These standardised tools provide an objective assessment based on pre-established criteria. Examples include:
  • The Allergy Quality of Life Questionnaire (AQLQ) for allergies.
  • The Quality of Life Questionnaire for Immunodeficient Patients (QoL-PID).
2. Physical assessment :
  • Measuring the impact of symptoms on the patient's daily activities.
  • Assess the frequency and severity of allergic or infectious episodes.
3. Emotional assessment :
  • Discuss the feelings of fear, anxiety, depression or isolation that may accompany these conditions.
  • Assess the patient's level of stress in relation to their illness and its implications.

4. Social impact :
- Examine how the condition affects the patient's ability to participate in social activities, school or work.
- Discuss any difficulties encountered in interpersonal relationships as a result of the illness.

5. Functional assessment :
- To determine the extent to which the condition limits the patient's ability to carry out everyday tasks, such as dressing, eating or getting around.

6. Satisfaction with care :
- Evaluate patient satisfaction with medical care, treatment and communication with healthcare professionals.

7. Economic aspects :
- Understand how the disease affects the patient's financial situation, in terms of treatment costs, days off work and other financial factors.

8. Educational aspects :
- Assess the patient's understanding of their condition, the treatments available and how they can manage their illness on a day-to-day basis.

9. Feedback from family and friends :
- Sometimes, obtaining information from family members or close friends can give a different perspective on how the disease affects the patient's life.

10. Regular monitoring :
- Quality of life assessment should not be a one-off event. It should be carried out regularly to monitor the patient's progress, adjust treatments and ensure that the patient's changing needs are taken into account.

Assessing the quality of life of allergic and immunocompromised patients is essential to providing holistic and personalised care. This not only addresses the physical symptoms, but also the emotional, social and functional challenges that patients may face. A multi-dimensional approach, combined with active and empathetic listening, ensures optimal care and enhances the patient's overall well-being.

Action to improve patient well-being

Improving the well-being of patients, particularly those suffering from allergies or immunological conditions, requires a comprehensive approach that encompasses the treatment of physical symptoms, psychological support and consideration of social and environmental aspects. Here are some interventions that can help improve the well-being of these patients:

1. Medical interventions :
   - **Optimising treatment**: Ensuring that the patient receives the most appropriate treatment for their condition, adjusting regularly as necessary.
   - **Therapeutic education**: educating patients about their disease, treatments and how best to manage their symptoms.
   - **Prevention**: Suggest appropriate vaccines and other measures to prevent infections in immunocompromised patients.
2. Psychological support :
   - **Individual therapy**: This can help to manage anxiety, depression or any other psychological problems associated with the disease.
   - **Support groups**: These can provide a platform for sharing experiences and getting emotional support.
   - **Relaxation techniques**: Meditation, mindfulness and other techniques can help manage stress.
3. Education and awareness :
   - **Educational workshops**: Organising workshops to help patients understand their condition and how to manage it.

- **Raising public awareness**: Making the general public more aware of the challenges faced by people with allergies or immunodeficiency can help them integrate into society.

4. Adapting to the environment :
   - Advise on home modifications to reduce allergens, such as the use of anti-dust mite covers, air purification, etc.
   - Promoting workspaces adapted for those with severe allergies.

5. Social intervention :
   - Facilitating access to services such as home support or rehabilitation services.
   - Offer professional reintegration programmes for those who have had to interrupt their career because of their illness.

6. Nutrition :
   - Offer dietary advice to avoid food allergens and promote a balanced diet.
   - Encourage eating habits that support the immune system.

7. Physical activity :
   - Encourage appropriate regular physical activity, which can boost general well-being and improve the immune system.

8. Additional interventions :
   - **Complementary therapies**: such as acupuncture, aromatherapy or massage therapy, which can help improve well-being.
   - **Integrative medicine**: Combining conventional and alternative treatments for a holistic approach.

9. Regular monitoring :
   - Regular visits with the GP or specialist nurse to assess how the disease is progressing and adjust interventions.

10. Use of technology :
   - Offer digital applications or platforms for monitoring symptoms, taking medication or telemedicine.

Improving patients' well-being requires a multi-dimensional, patient-centred approach. By understanding each patient's individual needs and proposing targeted interventions, it is possible to improve their quality of life and help them to manage their condition effectively.

Long-term monitoring and considerations for a normal life

Long-term monitoring of patients with allergies or immune disorders is essential to ensure optimum quality of life. Living with such conditions often requires adjustments, but with appropriate management, most patients can lead as normal a life as possible. Here are some key points to consider for long-term monitoring and to promote a normal life:

1. Regular medical consultations :
   - Routine visits enable the progress of the disease to be monitored, treatments to be adjusted and any complications to be detected.
2. Continuing education :
   - Patients must be regularly informed of the latest discoveries and recommendations concerning their condition.
   - Learning the warning signs of an exacerbation or allergic reaction can help with early intervention.
3. Self-management :
   - Self-management skills, such as recognising allergy triggers or managing medication, are crucial.
4. Psychosocial support :
   - Living with allergies or immunodeficiency can have an impact on mental health. Access to psychological support, whether through therapy or support groups, is essential.

5. Social integration :
  - Encourage participation in social, sporting and cultural activities, while taking the necessary precautions.
  - Raising awareness of the patient's specific needs among family and friends, teachers and employers.
6. Emergency action plan :
  - All patients at risk of serious reactions, such as anaphylaxis, should have a clearly defined emergency action plan, shared with those around them.
7. Healthy lifestyle :
  - A balanced diet, regular exercise and adequate sleep can improve general well-being and boost the immune system.
8. Specific precautions :
  - For example, patients with food allergies need to learn to read labels carefully, while those with environmental allergies may need to adjust their homes.
9. Care transitions :
  - Ensuring a smooth transition from paediatric to adult care.
10. Adherence to treatment :
  - Use reminders, apps or other tools to ensure that medication is taken as prescribed.
11. Networking :
  - Connecting patients to associations or support groups specific to their condition can provide a valuable source of advice and camaraderie.
12. Professional and academic considerations :
  - Depending on the severity of their condition, some patients may require accommodation at work or school.
13. Travel and leisure :
  - Patients should be informed about the precautions to be taken when travelling, such as taking extra medication or checking medical facilities at their destination.

The aim of long-term care is to enable patients to live as normal a life as possible, despite the challenges of their condition. This requires close collaboration between carers, patients, their families and society as a whole to create an environment in which patients can thrive while managing their health.

Challenges and successes of patient stories

The stories of patients with allergies or immune disorders can vary considerably depending on their individual experience, their state of health, their environment and their medical care. Each story is unique, but they often share common challenges as well as moments of success and hope. Here are just a few of the challenges and successes that are frequently encountered:

Challenges :

Diagnosis: Some patients can go for years without a precise diagnosis, which can lead to frustration and complications.

Stigmatisation and misunderstanding: People with food allergies or other conditions may find their problems misunderstood or minimised by those around them or by society as a whole.

Daily restrictions: Avoiding common allergens or managing a weakened immune system can lead to restrictions in daily life, ranging from diet to participation in certain activities.

Side effects of treatments : Medicines and other interventions can have troublesome or serious side effects.

Psychological support: Living with a chronic illness can have repercussions on mental health, including stress, anxiety and depression.

Medical costs: Medical consultations, treatments and procedures can be expensive, putting financial pressure on patients.

Successes and moments of hope :

Obtaining a diagnosis: For many people, receiving a precise diagnosis is a relief because it gives a direction for treatment.

Finding an effective treatment: Finding a treatment or intervention that works can considerably improve quality of life.

Support communities: Support groups and online communities can be a valuable source of advice, camaraderie and understanding.

Education and awareness: Educating relatives and the community broadens understanding and sympathy for the condition.

Moments of normality: Whether it's eating a food without an allergic reaction thanks to immunotherapy treatment, or taking part in an activity without worrying about exposure to an allergen, these moments when the disease doesn't define their existence are precious for patients.

Contributions to research: Some patients choose to take part in clinical trials, making a valuable contribution to the advancement of medicine and the discovery of new treatments.

Inspirational stories: Many patients use their experiences to educate, inspire and support others, whether through blogs, conferences or volunteering.

The challenges and successes of allergology and immunology patients highlight the resilience, courage and determination shown by many people in the face of health adversity. Their stories can inspire and educate others, and reinforce the importance of careful medical management and ongoing research in these fields.

Chapter 25:
GENETIC ASPECTS
AND ALLERGOLOGY AND IMMUNOLOGY

Genetics of allergies
and immunodeficiencies

Genetics play an important role in predisposing people to allergies and immunodeficiencies. Although the environment and other factors also play a role, studies have shown that genetics can increase the risk of developing these conditions. Here is an overview of the links between genetics, allergies and immunodeficiencies:

Genetics and allergies :

Atopy: Atopy is a genetic predisposition to developing allergies. If one or both parents are atopic (i.e. have a history of asthma, allergic rhinitis or eczema), the risk of their child developing an allergy is increased.

Polymorphisms: Research has identified specific polymorphisms (genetic variations) associated with an increased risk of allergies. These polymorphisms can affect the way the immune system recognises and responds to allergens.

Twin studies: Studies of monozygotic (identical) twins have shown a higher concordance of allergies than dizygotic (fraternal) twins, suggesting a strong genetic component.

Genetics and immunodeficiencies :

Primary immune deficiencies (PIDs): These deficiencies are generally caused by inherited genetic mutations that affect the development or function of the immune system. There are over 300 different types of PID identified, many of which are associated with specific genetic mutations.

Hereditary transmission: The modes of transmission of DIP can be autosomal recessive, autosomal dominant or X-linked. Understanding the mode of inheritance helps clinicians to advise families on the risk to other family members or future children.

Genetic counselling: Genetic counselling is often recommended for families with a history of DIP in order to assess the risk to current and future family members and to provide information on family planning and treatment options.

Challenges and ongoing research :
Technological advances, in particular next-generation genomic sequencing, are making it possible to discover new genes associated with allergies and PIDs. These discoveries can help to :

Understanding the underlying mechanisms of allergies and PIDs.

Identify individuals at risk before symptoms appear.

Develop new treatments targeting the underlying genetic causes.

Although the environment, exposure to allergens and other factors play a role in the development of allergies and immunodeficiencies, genetics is a key component. Research continues to expand our understanding of genetic links, offering new perspectives for the diagnosis, prevention and treatment of these conditions.

Genetic counselling for families

Genetic counselling is a process that helps individuals or families understand the risks of genetic diseases. It aims to inform and guide people about the implications, nature, prevention, screening and diagnosis of genetic conditions. Here is an overview of genetic counselling for families:

Objectives of genetic counselling :

Education: Providing detailed information about the disease or genetic condition in question.

Risk assessment: Estimating the risk of developing or transmitting a genetic disease.

Guidance: Helping people to make informed decisions about screening, management and family planning.

Support: Providing emotional support to individuals or families faced with the diagnosis or risk of a genetic disease.

Genetic counselling process :

Collecting medical history: Gathering detailed information on medical and family history to assess genetic risk.

Interpretation of history: Analysis of the information gathered to identify patterns or risks of genetic disease.

Education: Explanation of how the disease is transmitted, its prevalence, symptoms, and screening and treatment options.

Discussion of implications: Exploration of the implications of the genetic risk for the individual, their children or other family members.

Decision-making: Discussion of the different options available, such as genetic testing, medical monitoring, preventive interventions or procreation decisions.

Psychological support: Helping to manage stress, fear, guilt or other emotions associated with a genetic risk.

Genetic testing :

- These tests can confirm a diagnosis, estimate the risk of developing a disease or determine the risk of transmission to offspring.
- The genetic counsellor provides information on the benefits, risks and limitations of genetic testing.

The challenges of genetic counselling :

- **Complexity of information**: Genetics can be complex, and it can be difficult for some individuals or families to fully understand the implications.
- **Strong emotions**: Learning that you carry a gene predisposing you to a disease can provoke strong emotional reactions.
- **Difficult decisions**: Some people may be faced with difficult decisions concerning screening, prevention or procreation.

Genetic counselling is a valuable tool to help individuals and families understand and manage the risks associated with genetic conditions. An empathetic, informative and patient-centred approach is essential to support people through this often complex and emotional process.

Technological advances and genetic testing

Technological advances have revolutionised the field of genetic testing, enabling unprecedented discoveries and clinical applications. Here is an overview of the major innovations and impacts in this field:

1. Next-generation sequencing (NGS) :

- **Description**: NGS makes it possible to sequence millions of DNA fragments simultaneously.
- **Impact**: This has made the sequencing of the human genome much faster and cheaper, paving the way for

more accessible genetic tests and more in-depth analyses.

2. Genetic panels :

   Description: Rather than testing a single gene at a time, genetic panels test several genes simultaneously, generally linked to a condition or group of conditions.

   Impact: Panels make it possible to identify mutations in rare or unexpected conditions, improving diagnosis and treatment.

3. Direct-to-consumer genetic testing :

   Description: These tests, such as those offered by 23andMe or AncestryDNA, enable consumers to send a saliva sample to obtain genetic information without going to a healthcare professional.

   Impact: They have popularised genetics among the general public, although their clinical usefulness is sometimes open to debate.

4. CRISPR-Cas9 :

   Description: A genomic modification technology that can be used to specifically target and modify DNA segments in the genome.

   Impact: It has the potential to treat genetic diseases by targeting and correcting the mutations that cause the disease.

5. Pharmacogenetics :

   Description: The study of how an individual's genes influence their response to drugs.

   Impact: It enables personalised medicine, where treatments can be tailored to an individual's genetic make-up to maximise efficacy and minimise side effects.

6. Bioinformatics :

   Description: The use of software and mathematical tools to interpret and analyse genetic data.

Impact: Bioinformatics is essential for processing and interpreting the massive quantities of data generated by techniques such as NGS.
7. Non-invasive prenatal tests :
  Description: Tests that use a simple maternal blood sample to test circulating foetal DNA for certain genetic conditions.
  Impact: They offer a less risky option than invasive methods such as amniocentesis.

Challenges and ethical considerations :
Despite the advances, there are still challenges and ethical concerns associated with genetic testing, including :
  Privacy and confidentiality of genetic data.
  Possible genetic discrimination.
  The way in which information is communicated to patients.
  The interpretation of genetic variants of unknown significance.
  The psychological implications of a genetic diagnosis.

Technological advances have transformed the field of genetic testing, opening up new opportunities for the diagnosis, treatment and prevention of disease. However, these advances are also accompanied by significant challenges that need to be addressed in an ethical and responsible manner.

Ethics and social implications genetics in allergology

Ethics in genetics, particularly in the field of allergology, is of crucial importance as genetic information can have profound implications not only for the individual concerned, but also for his or her family and society as a whole. Here are some of the ethical issues and social implications associated with genetics in allergology:

1. Confidentiality and privacy :
    Genetic information is extremely personal. It is crucial to ensure that this data is protected and not disclosed without the patient's consent.
2. Genetic discrimination :
    There is a legitimate concern that genetic information can be used to discriminate against individuals, whether in employment, insurance or other areas. Some countries have passed laws to protect against this form of discrimination.
3. Informed consent :
    Before undergoing genetic testing, patients must be fully informed of the implications, risks and potential benefits. They must understand the possible consequences of discovering a genetic predisposition to an allergy or other condition.
4. Information for the family :
    If an individual is found to carry a genetic mutation that predisposes them to a severe allergy, this has implications for close relatives who may also be at risk. How, when and to whom to communicate this information becomes a complex ethical issue.
5. Genetic testing of children :
    Should children be tested for genetic predisposition to allergies, especially if no intervention is possible before adulthood? The psychological and social consequences of such information must be carefully weighed.
6. Psychosocial implications :
    The discovery of a genetic predisposition can have repercussions on self-esteem and personal identity, and can lead to anxiety or stress.
7. Genetic treatment guidelines :
    If an individual has a genetic predisposition to an allergy, could this influence treatment

recommendations, such as avoiding certain therapies or preferring certain interventions? And if so, what are the ethical implications of such a practice?

8. Marketing of genetic tests :

With the rise of direct-to-consumer genetic testing, how can we ensure that these tests are accurate, reliable and used ethically?

9. Equity and access :

Access to genetic testing and subsequent treatment may vary according to resources, geographical location or other socio-economic factors. How can equity of access to these vital resources be guaranteed?

The intersection of genetics and allergology offers exciting opportunities to improve patient care. However, it also raises important ethical issues that need to be carefully considered and addressed to ensure that these advances benefit everyone and respect the rights and dignity of individuals.

Chapter 26:
SKIN MANIFESTATIONS IN ALLERGOLOGY

Urticaria and angioedema

Urticaria and angioedema are two skin manifestations linked to the release of histamine and other inflammatory mediators in the dermis. These conditions can occur together or separately.

Hives

Definition

Hives are characterised by the sudden appearance of raised, red, itchy patches, often surrounded by an area of erythema. These plaques, known as urticarial papules, can vary in size and shape.

Causes

Urticaria can be triggered by a variety of factors, including :

- Allergic reactions (food, medication, insect stings)
- Contact with certain substances (latex, nettles)
- Physical conditions (pressure, cold, heat, sun, exercise)
- Infections (viral, bacterial, parasitic)
- Stress
- Certain diseases (lupus, certain cancers, thyroid disease)
- In many cases, the exact cause has not been identified.

Types

- **Acute urticaria**: lasts less than 6 weeks, generally due to a specific cause.
- **Chronic hives**: last for more than 6 weeks, often with no identifiable cause.

Angioedema

Angioedema is a deeper inflammation of the skin, often associated with urticaria. It manifests as sudden swelling of the deeper layers of the skin, particularly around the eyes and lips, as well as on the hands, feet and throat.

Causes

Triggers are similar to those for urticaria and can include allergic reactions, medication (e.g. ACE inhibitors) and hereditary factors.

Risks

Angioedema can be dangerous if it causes swelling of the throat, obstructing the airways.

Treatment

Treatment for urticaria and angioedema is aimed at relieving symptoms and avoiding identified triggers. Antihistamines are often prescribed to reduce itching and inflammation. In severe cases, oral corticosteroids may be necessary. For angioedema associated with respiratory problems, urgent medical intervention is essential.

Hives and angioedema are common conditions that can have a significant impact on an individual's quality of life. Understanding the potential triggers, symptoms and appropriate treatment is essential to effectively manage these conditions. In the event of persistent or severe symptoms, medical advice is recommended.

Atopic dermatitis and eczema

Atopic dermatitis (often called atopic eczema) is a chronic skin condition that can cause itching and inflammation of the skin. It is part of a group of allergic conditions that also includes asthma, allergic rhinitis and urticaria. The term "eczema" is often used interchangeably with "atopic dermatitis", although it actually refers to a broader group of inflammatory dermatological conditions.

Atopic dermatitis

Symptoms :
- Redness
- Intense itching
- Dry, scaly or rough skin
- Small bumps or vesicles, which may ooze or form scabs
- Inflammation and swelling
- Pigmentation (often in people with darker skin)

Causes and triggers :

The exact cause of atopic dermatitis is unknown, but it is probably due to a combination of genetic and environmental factors. Common triggers include:
- Allergens (pollens, dust mites, moulds, animals)
- Irritants (soaps, detergents, perfumes)
- Climatic variations (cold or drought)
- Stress
- Skin infections

Treatment :

Treatment aims to reduce itching, prevent flare-ups and moisturise the skin.
- Moisturisers and emollients
- Topical corticosteroids to reduce inflammation
- Antihistamines to control itching
- Immunosuppressive drugs in severe cases
- Light-based therapies (phototherapy)
- Avoiding known triggers

Eczema

Although the term "eczema" is often used to describe atopic dermatitis, it actually refers to a group of inflammatory skin conditions that also include :
- **Contact dermatitis**: caused by contact with irritants or allergens.

- **Nummular (or discoid) eczema:** characterised by round, scaly patches.
- **Dyshidrotic eczema**: small blisters on the hands and feet.
- **Seborrhoeic eczema**: red patches with yellowish scales, often on the scalp or face.

Atopic dermatitis and other forms of eczema can have a significant impact on quality of life. While there is no definitive cure, many treatment options are available to manage symptoms. It is essential to work closely with a dermatologist or allergist to establish a personalised treatment plan.

Skin tests:
techniques and interpretation

Skin tests are commonly used in allergology to determine whether a person is allergic to a specific substance. These tests involve introducing a small quantity of the suspected allergen into the skin and observing the reaction.

Skin testing techniques :
- **Prick** (or puncture) **test** :
  - A drop containing the allergen is placed on the skin, usually on the forearm or back.
  - The skin under the drop is gently pricked with a small needle or lancet.
  - If an allergic reaction occurs, a papule (elevation of the skin) surrounded by a reddish area will appear within 15 to 20 minutes.
- Intradermal test :
  - A small quantity of the allergen is injected directly into the dermis using a fine syringe.
  - This method is more sensitive than the prick test, but it is also more likely to produce false

positive reactions. It is often used to test for allergies to drugs or insect venoms.

Patch test :

Allergens are applied to patches which are then stuck to the skin, usually on the back.

These patches are generally left in place for 48 hours, after which they are removed and a first reading is taken. A second reading is often taken 72 to 96 hours after application.

It is used to diagnose allergic contact dermatitis.

Interpretation of results :

Positive reaction: appearance of a papule, often accompanied by redness and itching. The size of the papule is often measured. A larger reaction suggests greater sensitivity, but this does not necessarily predict the severity of symptoms in the event of actual exposure to the allergen.

Negative reaction: no papules or redness. This suggests that the patient is not sensitised to the allergen tested.

Questionable or false positive reaction: a small reaction that may be due to factors other than the allergy, such as irritation.

False negative reaction: absence of reaction even though the patient is allergic. This can occur if the patient is taking antihistamines or if the test is not carried out correctly.

Precautions:

Certain medications, particularly antihistamines, can interfere with skin tests and should be stopped before the test, as recommended by your doctor.

Skin tests should not be carried out during a flare-up of severe eczema or if the patient has recently had an anaphylactic reaction.

Skin tests are a valuable tool for identifying the allergens responsible for allergic symptoms. However, they must be carried out and interpreted by a specialist trained in allergology to obtain accurate results and avoid complications.

Treatment and care
skin manifestations

Allergic skin conditions such as urticaria, atopic dermatitis (eczema) and contact dermatitis require targeted management to control symptoms, prevent exacerbations and improve patients' quality of life. Here is an overview of the treatment and management of these conditions:

1. Urticaria :
   Antihistamines: These are the mainstay of treatment. Second-generation antihistamines, such as cetirizine, fexofenadine and loratadine, are preferred because they cause less drowsiness.
   Oral corticosteroids: Used for severe outbreaks of urticaria, but long-term use is avoided due to side effects.
   Omalizumab: A monoclonal antibody used to treat chronic spontaneous urticaria that does not respond to antihistamines.
2. Atopic dermatitis (Eczema) :
   Moisturising: Regular application of emollients helps repair the skin barrier and prevent dryness.
   Topical corticosteroids: These are used to reduce inflammation. The strength of the steroid is chosen according to the severity of the eczema.
   Topical calcineurin inhibitors: Tacrolimus and pimecrolimus may be used in cases of intolerance or resistance to corticosteroids.

Dupilumab: A monoclonal antibody used in the treatment of moderate to severe atopic dermatitis in adults and certain adolescents.

Phototherapy: Controlled UVB exposure to treat severe eczema.

3. Contact dermatitis :

Avoiding the allergen: Once the allergen has been identified by a patch test, the patient should avoid all contact with it.

Topical corticosteroids: Used to reduce inflammation.

Moist compresses: Help reduce inflammation and relieve symptoms.

General measures :

Patient education: Patients should be informed about the nature of their condition, potential triggers and how to manage and prevent flare-ups.

Avoid irritants: Perfumes, dyes, certain soaps and detergents can aggravate skin symptoms. Use hypoallergenic, fragrance-free products.

Controlling itching: Keeping nails short, using antihistamines and avoiding triggers can help control itching.

Psychotherapy: Stress can be a trigger for certain skin conditions. Managing stress through meditation, relaxation or psychotherapy can be beneficial.

The management of skin disorders often requires a multidisciplinary approach involving dermatologists, allergists, specialist nurses and other healthcare professionals.

Chapter 27:
NEW TARGETED THERAPIES

Monoclonal antibodies in allergology

Monoclonal antibodies (mAbs) are molecules designed to specifically target a single protein. In the field of allergology, they are used to target and neutralise key molecules involved in the allergic response. These drugs offer a targeted approach to the treatment of certain allergies and associated diseases, particularly when standard treatments are ineffective or poorly tolerated.

Some monoclonal antibodies used in allergology include:
Omalizumab (Xolair):

Target: Immunoglobulin E (IgE). By binding to IgE, omalizumab prevents it from attaching to mast cells and basophils, thereby reducing the release of histamine and other inflammatory mediators.

Indications: Moderate to severe allergic asthma, chronic spontaneous urticaria.

Dupilumab (Dupixent):

Target: Sub-units of interleukin 4 (IL-4) and IL-13 receptors, key cytokines involved in the inflammatory response of atopic dermatitis and asthma.

Indications: Moderate to severe atopic dermatitis, eosinophilic asthma, nasosinus polyposis.

Mepolizumab (Nucala), Reslizumab (Cinqair), Benralizumab (Fasenra):

Target: IL-5 or its receptor. IL-5 is essential for the survival and function of eosinophils, cells that play a key role in certain types of asthma.

Indications: Severe eosinophilic asthma.

Tezepelumab:

Target: Thymic stromal lymphopoietin (TSLP), an upstream cytokine that plays a role in initiating allergic inflammatory responses.

Indications: Severe, uncontrolled asthma.

Advantages of mAbs in allergology:

Targeted treatment: These treatments precisely target specific pathways involved in allergic pathology.

Durable response: Some patients may have a prolonged response even after stopping treatment.

Well tolerated: Fewer systemic side effects than other immunosuppressive treatments.

Limitations:

Cost: mAbs are generally expensive.

Route of administration: Most require administration by injection.

Variable responses: Not all patients respond to or benefit from therapy.

The availability and use of monoclonal antibodies in allergology has revolutionised the management of certain severe allergic diseases. As research progresses, other targets and monoclonal antibodies are likely to be identified and made available to treat an even wider range of allergic and immunological diseases.

Specific immunotherapy: recent advances

Specific immunotherapy (SIT) or allergen desensitisation is a therapeutic approach that has been used for over a century to treat certain allergies. It involves gradually administering increasing doses of a specific allergen to the patient, with the aim of modifying the immune response to this allergen and reducing or even eliminating symptoms on subsequent exposure.

Here are some recent advances in specific immunotherapy:
Sublingual STI (SLIT):

SLIT is an alternative to injectable immunotherapy (SCIT). It is administered in the form of tablets or drops under the tongue.

SLIT products have been approved for grass pollen, tree pollen, dust mites and other allergens.

STI for food allergies:

Studies have shown promising results for oral TSI (OIT) for allergies to milk, eggs, peanuts and other foods.

In 2020, the first OIT treatment for peanut allergy, Palforzia, was approved in the United States.

ITS combined:

For patients allergic to several pollens or allergens, treatments combining several allergens are being studied.

Protocol optimisation:

New approaches aimed at reducing the duration of SIT while increasing its efficacy and safety are being studied, such as high-dose SIT and ultra-rapid SIT.

Additives and new formulations:

Research is underway to improve the efficacy and safety of SIT by using adjuvants (compounds that boost the immune response) or by modifying the structure of allergens.

STI for severe asthma:

Although SIT is traditionally used for mild to moderate respiratory allergies, studies are underway to assess its effectiveness in more severe asthma patients.

Use of biotechnologies:

The development of modified allergoids (allergens modified in the laboratory to reduce their ability to provoke an allergic reaction while retaining the ability to induce an immune response) is underway.

Customised approaches:

With the growing understanding of the genetics and biology of allergies, personalised SIT approaches based on the patient's genetic or immunological profile are being studied.

SIT remains one of the few therapies capable of modifying the natural progression of allergic disease. With recent and future advances, its potential to treat a greater number of allergies and patients more effectively and safely is growing.

Gene therapies and stem cells for immunodeficiencies

Gene therapies and stem cell approaches have transformed the treatment of certain primary immunodeficiencies (PIDs), which are inherited disorders of the immune system. These advances offer the hope of treating, or even curing, some of these often debilitating and sometimes fatal disorders.

- Gene therapy:
    - **Principle**: Gene therapy aims to correct the defective gene that causes immunodeficiency. This is generally achieved by introducing a functional copy of the gene into the patient's cells.
    - **Applications**: Gene therapy has been most successful in the treatment of severe combined immunodeficiency (SCID), particularly X-linked SCID and SCID caused by ADA deficiency. Other SCIDs are also being investigated for gene therapy intervention.
    - **Methodology**: Typically, haematopoietic stem cells (which give rise to all blood cells) are taken from the patient, modified in the laboratory to introduce the correct gene, and then reinjected into the patient.
- Haematopoietic stem cell transplantation (HSCT):
    - **Principle**: HSCT aims to replace the patient's defective immune system with a healthy immune system, generally from a compatible donor.
    - **Applications**: HSCT has been successfully used to treat several types of PID, including SCID and chronic septic granulomatosis.
    - **Challenges**: The main difficulty with HSCT is finding a suitable donor. Even if there is a match, there is a risk of rejection or graft-versus-host disease (GVHD).
- Innovations and challenges:
    - **Safety**: Early gene therapy approaches were associated with a risk of inducing leukaemia. New techniques, such as the use of self-

inactivating viral vectors, have increased safety.

- **Genome editing**: Technologies such as CRISPR-Cas9 now make it possible to precisely target and correct the specific genetic mutations responsible for PDI.
- **Accessibility**: While these therapies offer revolutionary potential, their high cost and limited availability may make them inaccessible to all patients.

Gene and stem cell therapies offer immense potential for the treatment of primary immunodeficiencies. While many challenges remain, continued advances in these areas offer the hope of improved therapeutic options for patients with PID.

The future of treatment: research and innovation

The field of allergology and immunology is constantly evolving, with many innovations and research projects in progress. Here's a look at the trends, research and innovations that could shape the future of treatments in this field:

- **Personalised therapies**: With the advent of genomics and biotechnology, treatments can be increasingly tailored to the individual, enabling more targeted and effective interventions based on the patient's genetic and immunological profile.
- **Microbiome and immunology**: The microbiome, in particular the gut microbiome, is increasingly recognised as playing a key role in modulating the immune system. Future research could focus on

manipulating the microbiome to treat or prevent allergic and immunological diseases.

- **New-generation immunotherapy**: New methods of administration, such as skin patches or sublingual tablets, as well as immunotherapy for new allergens, are currently being developed.
- **Gene and cell therapies**: As mentioned above, these therapies offer the potential to treat or even cure certain primary immunodeficiencies.
- **Nanotechnology**: Nanotechnology could be used to target drugs more effectively, reducing side effects and increasing the effectiveness of treatments.
- **Artificial intelligence (AI) and predictive medicine**: AI could be used to analyse huge datasets, identify trends or patterns, and even predict the risk of allergies or immunodeficiencies in individuals.
- **Allergy vaccines**: Research is underway to develop vaccines that could prevent or reduce the severity of allergic reactions.
- **Biologics and small molecules**: Biological agents, such as monoclonal antibodies, and targeted small molecules continue to be developed to treat various allergic and immunological conditions.
- **Education and awareness**: With allergies on the rise worldwide, public awareness and education, as well as training for healthcare professionals, will be essential to prevent and manage these conditions.
- **Integrative approaches**: By recognising that patients are more than the sum of their symptoms, a holistic approach to care could integrate nutrition, psychology, physiotherapy and other disciplines.

The future of treatments in allergology and immunology is promising, with a combination of new technologies, innovative therapeutic approaches and a deeper understanding of the underlying mechanisms of disease.

The key will be to integrate these advances in a patient-centred way to provide the highest quality of care.

Chapter 28:
PSYCHOLOGICAL SUPPORT
AND SUPPORT

Psychological impact
chronic allergies

The psychological impact of chronic allergies is often underestimated. However, these conditions, like any chronic illness, can have a significant impact on a person's mental and emotional well-being. Here are a few aspects of this impact:

- **Anxiety and stress**: Fear of allergens, particularly in the case of severe allergies such as food allergy where accidental exposure can cause anaphylaxis, can cause constant anxiety. Allergy sufferers may also experience stress as they try to avoid exposure and manage their symptoms.
- **Social isolation**: Individuals with food allergies, for example, may avoid social outings where food is involved for fear of an allergic reaction. They may also feel excluded or misunderstood by their peers.
- **Self-esteem and body image**: Allergy symptoms, such as eczema or atopic dermatitis, can affect physical appearance, which can have an impact on self-esteem and body image.
- **Depression**: Ongoing allergy management, social isolation and daily challenges can lead to feelings of sadness, despair and even depression.
- **Fatigue**: Allergy symptoms, such as congestion or sneezing, can disrupt sleep, leading to chronic fatigue and reduced quality of life.

- **Impact on daily life**: Simple, everyday activities, such as eating out, choosing products in the supermarket or travelling, can become complex and stressful for allergy sufferers.
- **Emotional exhaustion**: The constant vigilance required to avoid allergens and manage symptoms can lead to emotional exhaustion.
- **Feelings of frustration**: Allergy sufferers may feel frustrated by persistent symptoms, despite their best efforts to manage them.
- **Impact on family members**: Parents of allergic children may feel anxious, guilty and stressed about their child's health and safety.

It is crucial for healthcare professionals to recognise and address these psychological aspects when caring for allergy sufferers. A comprehensive approach, incorporating psychological and educational interventions, can help patients and their families to better manage the emotional challenges associated with chronic allergies.

Managing stress and anxiety in patients

Managing stress and anxiety is an essential part of the overall management of patients, particularly those suffering from chronic illnesses such as allergies. Anxiety and stress can not only exacerbate physiological symptoms, but also reduce a patient's quality of life. Here are some strategies and approaches to help manage stress and anxiety in patients:

- **Therapeutic education**: Informing patients about their condition and treatment can reduce the anxiety associated with the unknown. A better understanding of their condition can help them feel more in control.

- **Cognitive behavioural therapies (CBT)**: CBT is a form of psychotherapy that helps individuals identify and change the negative thoughts and behaviours that may be contributing to their anxiety.
- **Relaxation techniques**: Methods such as deep breathing, meditation and progressive muscle relaxation can help reduce stress and anxiety.
- **Physical exercise**: Physical activity can reduce stress by releasing endorphins, which are natural painkillers, and helping people to turn away from their worries.
- **Group therapy**: Joining a support group where individuals can share their experiences and feelings can provide a safe space to express concerns and learn from others.
- **Complementary therapies**: Approaches such as acupuncture, yoga and massage therapy can help some people manage stress.
- **Time management**: Helping patients to organise their lives in such a way as to avoid overwork, take breaks and prioritise their activities can reduce stress.
- **Avoidance of stimulants**: Reducing or eliminating caffeine and other stimulants can help reduce anxiety in some people.
- **Specialist consultation**: In cases of severe anxiety, referral to a psychologist or psychiatrist may be necessary for further assessment and treatment.
- **Medication**: In some cases, anxiolytic or antidepressant medication may be prescribed to help manage anxiety. These drugs must be prescribed with caution and under medical supervision.
- **Planning and preparation**: For allergy sufferers, having a clear plan of action in the event of exposure to an allergen can reduce anxiety.
- **Biofeedback techniques**: These techniques teach patients how to control certain physiological functions to help reduce stress.

It is crucial to recognise that each individual is unique. What works for one person may not work for another. A personalised, holistic approach is therefore essential to effectively manage stress and anxiety in patients.

Support groups and self-help networks

Support groups and self-help networks play an essential role in the management of patients with chronic diseases, including allergies and immunodeficiencies. These groups provide a platform where patients, their families and loved ones can share experiences, exchange information and get emotional support. Here are the main features and benefits of these groups:

- **Emotional support**: Being heard and understood by people going through similar situations can alleviate feelings of isolation and stigmatisation. Simply knowing that you are not alone can have a profoundly beneficial impact on your emotional well-being.
- **Exchanging information**: Support groups often offer a wealth of information based on personal experience. Participants can share practical advice, tips and resources that have worked for them.
- **Education**: These groups often organise educational sessions with healthcare professionals to inform members about the latest medical advances, new therapies and best practice in disease management.
- **Advocates for change**: Support groups can also function as patient advocacy groups, campaigning for policy changes, better care and funding for research.
- **Social and leisure activities**: Many of these groups organise social events, outings or workshops that

offer a welcome escape from the daily routine of managing the disease.

- **Networking**: Groups enable patients and families to create strong support networks, which can be useful in times of need, such as during a crisis.
- **Strengthening resilience**: By sharing stories of successes, challenges overcome and lessons learned, members can inspire and strengthen the resilience of others.
- **Support for families and loved ones**: These groups also provide a platform for patients' families and loved ones, enabling them to understand the disease, learn how best to support their loved one and manage their own stress.
- **Links with healthcare professionals**: Some groups are affiliated to hospitals or clinics and can facilitate links with healthcare professionals for consultations, advice or treatment.
- **Online support**: With the advent of digital technologies, many support groups now offer online platforms, forums and discussion groups for those who cannot physically attend meetings.

By joining a support group or self-help network, patients can not only improve their quality of life, but also acquire skills and knowledge to help them manage their condition effectively. It is important to choose a group that meets the patient's specific needs, in a caring and respectful atmosphere.

Specific counselling techniques for allergology nurses

The role of the allergy nurse goes far beyond the simple administration of medical care. Allergy patients can often experience anxiety, stress or frustration related to their condition. Counselling by a nurse can help these patients to better understand, manage and live with their allergies. Here are some specific counselling techniques that allergy nurses can adopt:

- **Active listening**: Listening attentively to patients' concerns, fears and questions is essential. Not only does this provide important information for care, it also shows patients that they are being heard and understood.
- **Questioning techniques**: Ask open-ended questions to encourage patients to share their feelings and experiences. For example, "How do you feel about your allergy?" or "What challenges do you face on a daily basis because of your allergy?".
- **Validation of feelings**: Acknowledging and validating the patient's feelings can help strengthen the therapeutic bond and reduce anxiety.
- **Education**: Providing clear and understandable information about allergy, its causes, tests, treatments and preventive measures. This can help demystify the disease and give patients a sense of control.
- **Coping strategies**: Suggest strategies to help patients manage the stress or anxiety associated with their allergy, such as relaxation, meditation or keeping a diary.
- **Assertiveness techniques**: Encouraging patients to communicate openly with those around them about their allergies, to ask for help if necessary and to stand up for their needs.
- **Practical advice**: Offer suggestions on how to manage everyday situations, such as preparing meals to avoid allergens or managing social situations.
- **Role of games and scenarios**: This is particularly useful for children. Playing scenarios can help children understand their allergy and know how to

react in certain situations, such as when they are offered a food to which they are allergic.

- **Support groups**: Encourage participation in support groups or educational workshops where patients can share their experiences and learn from others.
- **Positive reinforcement**: Encourage and praise patients when they take steps to manage their allergy effectively, such as avoiding allergens or following a treatment plan.

It is important for the allergist nurse to receive regular training in counselling techniques and to keep up to date with the latest research and recommendations in the field of allergology. This will enable them to provide effective, evidence-based support to their patients.

Chapter 29:
DRUG ALLERGIES

Mechanisms and manifestations drug reactions

Drug reactions can vary considerably in severity and presentation. They are classified into several types, depending on their underlying mechanisms. Understanding these mechanisms is essential for making a correct diagnosis, avoiding future reactions and providing appropriate treatment.

1. Types of drug reactions:

Type I (Immediate reactions or immediate hypersensitivity) :

- Mechanism: These reactions are mediated by IgE antibodies that bind to a drug. On subsequent exposure, the drug binds to these IgE antibodies, triggering the release of histamine and other chemical mediators from mast cells and basophils.
- Manifestations: urticaria, angioedema, rhinitis, asthma, anaphylaxis.
- Examples of medicines: penicillin, cephalosporins.

Type II (Cytotoxicity) :

- Mechanism: Antibodies bind directly to a target cell, leading to its destruction.
- Symptoms: haemolytic anaemia, thrombocytopenia, agranulocytosis.
- Examples of medicines: penicillin, quinidine, methyl-dopa.

Type III (immune complex reactions) :

- Mechanism: Drug-antibody complexes are deposited in tissues, causing inflammation.
- Manifestations: fever, rash, arthralgia, glomerulonephritis.

- Examples of medicines: sulphonamides, penicillin, phenytoin.

Type IV (Delayed reactions or cell-mediated hypersensitivity) :
- Mechanism: Mediated by T lymphocytes, which are activated by the drug or its metabolites.
- Manifestations: contact dermatitis, maculopapular rash, drug fever.
- Examples of drugs: anticonvulsants, sulphonamides, allopurinol.

2. Other non-immunological drug reactions:
- **Drug intolerance**: similar to an allergic reaction, but without an immunological mechanism. For example, flushing caused by niacin.
- **Toxicity**: predictable, dose-dependent side effects, such as renal toxicity of aminoglycosides.
- **Idiosyncratic effects**: rare and unpredictable effects that are not dose-dependent. For example, aplastic anaemia induced by chloramphenicol.
- **Drug interactions**: when two or more drugs taken together cause an effect that does not occur when they are taken separately.

3. Diagnosis and management:
- A detailed medical history, including when the medication was taken, symptoms and their evolution.
- Skin tests can be useful for certain allergic drug reactions.
- Immediate management may include stopping the drug in question, providing symptomatic treatment (e.g. antihistamines for urticaria) and, in serious cases, emergency medical intervention (e.g. administration of epinephrine for anaphylaxis).

It is crucial for healthcare professionals to recognise drug reactions, differentiate them from other conditions and provide appropriate management to avoid potentially fatal complications.

Desensitisation protocols

Desensitisation, also known as tolerance-inducing immunotherapy, is a process by which a patient is gradually exposed to an allergenic or medicinal agent in order to increase the threshold of tolerance to that agent. This process is commonly used for drug allergies, particularly when there is an absolute need for a drug for which there is no suitable alternative.

Indications for desensitisation:
- Allergy to an essential drug for which there is no equivalent therapeutic alternative.
- Allergies to hymenoptera venoms to prevent future anaphylactic reactions.
- Certain food allergies, although this indication is still under study.

General desensitisation protocol:
- **Initial assessment:** Before starting desensitisation, a full assessment of the allergic reaction is necessary. This includes a detailed history of the reaction and, if possible, skin tests.
- **Controlled environment:** Desensitisation must always be carried out in a medical environment, where the equipment and medicines needed to manage an anaphylactic reaction are immediately available.
- **Progressive administration:** The drug or allergen is administered starting with a very low dose, which is gradually increased according to a predefined protocol. This may take place over several hours or days.

- **Continuous monitoring:** The patient is monitored continuously during the process to detect any adverse reactions.
- **Maintenance dose:** Once the therapeutic dose has been reached without a reaction, the drug can be administered according to the normal treatment schedule.

Some examples of specific protocols:

- **Desensitisation to antibiotics (e.g. penicillin):** The protocol begins with a very low, usually diluted, dose of the drug, which is doubled every 15 to 30 minutes until the therapeutic dose is reached.
- **Desensitisation to hymenoptera venom:** This procedure is generally carried out over a longer period, starting with an injection of very dilute venom, with gradual increases at defined intervals, until the maintenance dose is reached.
- **Aspirin desensitisation:** This protocol is often used in patients with nasal polyposis and aspirin-exacerbated asthma. It starts with a very low dose of aspirin, which is gradually increased to the desired dose.

Risks associated with desensitisation:

Despite all precautions, there is always a risk of allergic reaction during desensitisation. However, with close monitoring, these reactions are generally less serious than if the drug were administered in the normal dose without desensitisation.

Desensitisation is a powerful technique that allows allergy sufferers to be treated with essential medicines or allergens. It should always be carried out under the supervision of an allergist or trained healthcare professional.

Tips to avoid interactions and exhibitions

Avoiding interactions and exposure to potentially harmful allergens or medicines is essential to prevent adverse reactions. Here is some general advice, followed by specific recommendations depending on the type of allergen or medicine:

General advice:
- **Knowledge of allergens/medications:** Be aware of the substances to which you are allergic or intolerant.
- **Read labels:** Whether it's food, medication or cosmetics, always read labels carefully to spot the presence of a potential allergen.
- **Educate those around you:** Make sure your family, friends and colleagues know about your allergies to help prevent accidental exposure.
- **Wear a medical bracelet:** A medical bracelet or card can quickly inform healthcare professionals in the event of an emergency.
- **Have a plan of action:** Have a plan in case of accidental exposure, and always keep the necessary medication to hand (for example, an epinephrine auto-injector for severe allergies).

Specific advice:
- Food allergies:
  - Avoid restaurants where cross-contamination is likely.
  - When eating out, always tell the staff about your allergies.
  - Learn how to cook at home and prepare allergen-free meals.
- Drug allergies:
  - Inform all your healthcare providers of your allergies.

- When prescribing a new drug, check with the pharmacist for any interaction or similarity with an allergenic drug.
- Keep an up-to-date list of all your medicines and allergies so you can share it with others if the need arises.
- Allergies to insect bites:
  - Wear long-sleeved clothing and closed shoes when outdoors.
  - Avoid perfumes or scented lotions that attract insects.
  - Remain vigilant near nests or areas where insects are common.
- Allergies to pollen and other outdoor allergens:
  - Stay indoors on days with high pollen counts or during allergen peaks.
  - Use air filters in your home.
  - Shower after being outdoors to remove allergens from your skin and hair.
- Household allergies (dust mites, moulds, pets):
  - Use anti-dust mite covers for your bedding.
  - Keep humidity levels low in your home.
  - Vacuum regularly with a HEPA filter and clean your home frequently.
  - Avoid carpets, prefer hard floors.
- Drug reactions:
  - Be aware of the medicines and supplements you are taking and their potential interactions.
  - Always consult a healthcare professional before adding a new drug or supplement.

By following this advice and remaining informed and vigilant, you can considerably reduce the risk of unwanted exposure and interactions.

The nurse's role in monitoring and patient education

Nurses play a crucial role in patient care. Their role extends far beyond direct clinical care, encompassing education, advice, monitoring and care coordination. When it comes to allergology and immunology, here's how these functions manifest themselves:

1. Assessment and monitoring:
   - **Initial assessment:** The nurse assesses the patient's medical history, identifies signs and symptoms of allergies or immunodeficiency, and gathers information on potential triggers or recent exposures.
   - **Continuous monitoring:** The nurse regularly monitors the patient's condition, in particular vital signs, the appearance of new symptoms or the worsening of existing symptoms.
   - **Diagnostic tests:** The nurse may be involved in carrying out or interpreting skin tests or other diagnostic tests.
2. Patient education:
   - **Information on the disease:** Explain the nature of the allergy or immunodeficiency, its causes, symptoms and course.
   - **Managing medicines:** educating patients about the medicines prescribed, their mode of action, dosage, potential side effects and drug interactions.
   - **Avoiding triggers:** advising patients on how to avoid allergens or triggers, whether in food, the environment or medication.
   - **Emergency action plan:** Develop and teach an action plan for severe allergic reactions, including the use of an epinephrine auto-injector.

- **Self-care:** Encouraging and teaching patients how to manage their symptoms at home, for example through desensitisation or hygiene techniques.

3. Care coordination:

- **Liaison with other healthcare professionals:** The nurse works closely with doctors, pharmacists, dieticians, respiratory therapists and other healthcare professionals to ensure comprehensive care.
- **Discharge planning:** The nurse plays an essential role in discharge planning, ensuring that the patient has all the necessary medicines, equipment and instructions.

4. Emotional support:

- **Listening and support:** Offering a listening ear and providing emotional support to patients and their families in the face of the challenges posed by allergies or immunodeficiencies.
- **Referral:** If necessary, refer the patient to psychological support services or support groups.

The allergology and immunology nurse's training and experience make her a valuable resource for patients and their families. They not only provide quality care, but also education and support to help patients manage their disease effectively on a daily basis.

Chapter 30:
VACCINATIONS AND IMMUNOLOGY

Benefits and risks of vaccines for allergy sufferers

Vaccines are essential tools for preventing infectious diseases. However, as with any medical treatment, there are benefits and risks associated with their administration, particularly in allergy sufferers. Here is an overview of the benefits and risks of vaccination for this population:

Benefits :
- **Protection against disease**: Vaccines offer protection against potentially serious and sometimes fatal diseases.
- **Reduced transmission**: By protecting individuals against certain infections, vaccines also reduce the risk of transmission in the population, indirectly protecting those who are not vaccinated.
- **Preventing complications**: People with allergies may be more susceptible to certain complications of infectious diseases. Vaccination can reduce this risk.
- **Reduced use of antibiotics**: By preventing certain bacterial infections, vaccines can reduce the need to use antibiotics, thereby helping to combat antibiotic resistance.

Risks :
- **Allergic reactions to vaccine components**: Some individuals may be allergic to components present in vaccines, such as gelatine or preservatives. These allergic reactions are rare but can be serious.
- **Anaphylaxis**: Although very rare, an anaphylactic reaction is a serious complication that can occur after

vaccination. That's why it's essential that vaccination is carried out in an environment where anaphylaxis can be rapidly treated.

- **Local reactions**: Pain, swelling or redness at the injection site are common but usually mild and temporary.
- **Specific concerns**: People with a history of severe allergies, particularly to a component of a vaccine, should discuss the risks and benefits of vaccination with their allergist.

Recommendations:

- **Prior   consultation**: People with a history of severe allergies or allergic reactions to a previous vaccine should consult an allergist before vaccination.
- **Post-vaccination monitoring**: It is advisable to remain under surveillance for 15 to 30 minutes after vaccination, particularly if the individual has a history of severe allergies, in order to detect and rapidly treat any allergic reaction.
- **Information**: Patients should be made aware of the signs and symptoms of an allergic reaction so that they can seek medical help if necessary.
- **Vaccine alternatives**: In certain cases, if there is a risk of allergy to a specific component of a vaccine, an alternative version of the vaccine without this component may be available.

Although vaccines present risks for allergy sufferers, these risks are generally low, especially when compared with the significant benefits of vaccination. Open communication with healthcare professionals and prior assessment can help minimise these risks.

Vaccinations for immunocompromised patients

Vaccination in immunocompromised patients is an important issue because these patients are at increased risk of infection due to their weakened immune systems. However, the choice of vaccines, their timing and effectiveness may be different for this population compared with immunocompetent individuals. Here is an overview of vaccination in immunocompromised patients:

Types of immunodepression:
There are several types of immunodepression, including :
- Congenital or primary (such as primary immunodeficiencies).
- Acquired or secondary (such as HIV, immunosuppressive drugs, chemotherapy, etc.).

Live attenuated vaccines:
- Live attenuated vaccines contain live viruses or bacteria that have been modified so that they do not cause disease.
- They are generally **contraindicated** in immunocompromised patients because of the risk of infection.
- Examples: MMR (measles, mumps and rubella), BCG, shingles vaccine, oral polio vaccine, etc.

Inactivated vaccines:
- These vaccines contain viruses or bacteria that have been killed or fragments of these pathogens.
- They are **generally safe** for immunocompromised patients.
- However, their efficacy may be reduced in these patients.
- Examples: vaccines against influenza, inactivated polio, hepatitis B, etc.

Specific recommendations:
- **Before planned immunosuppression**: If possible, vaccinate patients before the start of planned immunosuppression (for example, before transplantation or chemotherapy). This gives a better chance of an effective immune response.
- **Avoid live vaccines**: When the patient is already immunocompromised, live vaccines should be avoided unless the benefit clearly outweighs the risk.
- **Monitoring antibody titres**: In some cases, it may be useful to check antibody titres after vaccination to assess the immune response.
- **Vaccination of contacts**: Vaccinate family members and other close contacts to reduce the risk of exposure to the immunocompromised patient. This creates a "shield" around the patient.

Other considerations:
- **Foreseeable illnesses**: In certain situations, such as before a splenectomy, vaccination against specific infections (such as pneumococcus) is recommended.
- **Specialist consultation**: It is crucial to consult a specialist in immunology or infectious diseases for specific recommendations on vaccinating immunocompromised patients.

Vaccination of immunocompromised patients is essential to prevent infections. However, their vaccination plan must be carefully designed according to the nature and degree of immunosuppression, the risks associated with specific vaccines and the risk of exposure to pathogens.

Managing reactions allergic to vaccines

The management of allergic reactions to vaccines is essential to ensure patient safety while maintaining public confidence in vaccination programmes. Although rare, allergic reactions to vaccines can occur and must be managed quickly and effectively.

Recognition of allergic reactions:
- Immediate reactions:
    - Hives or rash
    - Swelling of the face, lips or throat
    - Difficulty breathing or wheezing
    - Feeling unwell or weak
    - Increased heart rate
    - Lower blood pressure
- Delayed reactions:
    - Skin rash, fever or joint pain occurring several days after vaccination.

Prevention of allergic reactions:
- Detailed medical history:
    - Before vaccination, ask the patient about any history of allergies, in particular allergic reactions to previous vaccines or their components.
- Know the components of the vaccine:
    - Some patients may be allergic to specific components of vaccines, such as gelatine, residual antibiotics or preservatives. Knowing what these components are helps you choose the right vaccine.
- Monitoring after vaccination:
    - It is usual to monitor patients for 15 minutes after vaccination. People with a history of severe allergic reactions to a vaccine or one of its components should be monitored for 30 minutes.

Managing allergic reactions:
- Stop administering the vaccine:
    - If a reaction occurs during administration, stop immediately.
- Call for emergency medical assistance:

- If symptoms are severe, such as anaphylaxis, call the emergency services immediately.
- Administration of epinephrine (adrenaline):
  - For severe reactions, epinephrine is the treatment of choice. It should be administered intramuscularly into the anterolateral thigh muscle.
- Surveillance:
  - Monitor the patient closely for signs of worsening or improvement.
- Other treatments:
  - Antihistamines and corticosteroids can be used to manage less severe symptoms, but they do not replace epinephrine for severe reactions.
- Report:
  - Document the reaction and inform the patient's primary care provider. In addition, report the reaction through national vaccine adverse reaction monitoring systems.
- Subsequent assessment:
  - Patients who have had an allergic reaction to a vaccine should be assessed by an allergist to determine the exact cause and to decide on the safety of subsequent administrations of the vaccine or similar vaccines.

Most allergic reactions to vaccines are mild, but rapid and appropriate management is essential in the event of a severe reaction. Good communication with patients about the risks and benefits, and preparation for the management of allergic reactions, are essential to ensure patient safety and maintain confidence in vaccination programmes.

The nurse's role in education and promoting vaccination

Nurses play an essential role in educating and promoting vaccination. Their actions are crucial to ensuring optimal vaccination coverage, preventing infectious diseases and guaranteeing public health. Here are the nurse's main responsibilities and actions in this area:

- Patient and public education :
    - To provide information on the importance of vaccination, the diseases that can be prevented, and the benefits and potential risks involved.
    - Debunking myths and misconceptions about vaccines, often spread by social media or rumours.
    - Reassure hesitant parents by addressing their concerns and providing evidence-based information.
- Assessment of health and vaccination history :
    - Review medical records to determine which vaccinations are required according to age, state of health and local/national recommendations.
    - Identify potential contraindications to vaccination.
- Administration of vaccines :
    - Ensuring correct and safe administration techniques.
    - Monitor patients after vaccination to detect any adverse reactions.
- Documentation:
    - Keep patient vaccination records up to date.
    - Document any adverse reactions and report serious adverse events to the relevant health authorities.

- Community awareness :
    - Taking part in vaccination campaigns in the community, particularly in schools, community health centres and at special events.
    - Working with other health professionals to reinforce messages about the importance of vaccination.
- Continuous updating :
    - Keep up to date with the latest vaccine recommendations, new research and best practice in vaccination.
    - Participate in ongoing training to ensure evidence-based practice.
- Managing vaccine hesitations :
    - Identify hesitant patients or families and start an open, non-confrontational dialogue to understand their concerns.
    - Provide clear, accurate, evidence-based information to help inform the decision.
- Advocacy :
    - Working with decision-makers, public health bodies and other health professionals to promote vaccination policies.
    - Engage in advocacy initiatives to reinforce the importance of vaccination and address barriers to vaccination coverage.
- Emergency management :
    - In the context of epidemic outbreaks, the nurse can play a key role in the rapid implementation of vaccination campaigns to control the spread of the disease.

Nurses are central to the promotion of vaccination, playing educational, clinical, administrative and advocacy roles. Their ability to educate, reassure and care for patients makes them an essential element in ensuring public health through vaccination.

Chapter 31:
INDOOR ENVIRONMENTAL ASPECTS

Common allergens
of the indoor environment:
dust mites, mould, animal hair

Allergens in the indoor environment can cause a range of symptoms in sensitive individuals, from mild irritation to severe allergic reactions. Here is a detailed description of common indoor allergens:

- Mites :
  - **Description**: These are tiny arachnids that live in house dust. They feed mainly on dead human skin cells.
  - **Main sources**: Mattresses, pillows, duvets, carpets, curtains, plush and other textiles.
  - **Common symptoms**: Sneezing, nasal congestion, itchy eyes, asthma, skin rashes.
  - **Prevention**: Use anti-dust mite covers for mattresses and pillows, wash bedding regularly at high temperatures, keep humidity levels low, vacuum frequently with a HEPA-filtered hoover.
- Mould :
  - **Description**: Moulds are microscopic fungi that grow in conditions of high humidity.
  - **Main sources**: Bathrooms, cellars, kitchens, plant pots, refrigerators, windows and areas where water stagnates.
  - **Common symptoms**: Sneezing, nasal congestion, coughing, asthma, eye irritation, skin rashes.

- **Prevention**: Maintain good ventilation, use a dehumidifier if necessary, regularly clean damp areas with an antifungal product, eliminate water leaks.
- Animal hair :
  - **Description: These are not** just hairs, but also scales (dead skin), saliva, urine and secretions from animals' sebaceous glands.
  - **Main sources**: Domestic animals such as cats, dogs, birds and rodents.
  - **Common symptoms**: Sneezing, nasal congestion, asthma, itchy eyes, skin rashes.
  - **Prevention**: If possible, avoid having pets if you are allergic. Otherwise, bathe your pet regularly, vacuum frequently, keep pets out of bedrooms, use air purifiers, and wash your pet's bedding and toys regularly.

It is essential to recognise these sources of allergens in the indoor environment and take steps to reduce them. For sensitive individuals, a significant reduction in exposure can lead to an improvement in symptoms and a better quality of life.

Tips for reducing exposure to household allergens

Reducing exposure to household allergens can help prevent or alleviate allergic symptoms. Here are a few tips for minimising exposure to these allergens in your home:

- Mites :
  - Use anti-dust mite covers for mattresses, pillows and duvets.
  - Regularly wash bedding at a high temperature (at least 60°C).

- Vacuum frequently with a hoover fitted with a HEPA (High Efficiency Particulate Air) filter.
  - Avoid rugs or carpets in bedrooms.
  - Keep humidity levels low, ideally between 30% and 50%.
  - Air the rooms regularly.
- Mould :
  - Ensure good ventilation in damp rooms such as bathrooms and kitchens.
  - Use a dehumidifier in damp areas.
  - Clean surfaces regularly with antifungal products.
  - Eliminate all sources of water leaks quickly.
  - Avoid over-watering houseplants.
- Animal hair and dander :
  - If possible, choose animals with a reputation for producing fewer allergens (although no animal is completely hypoallergenic).
  - Restrict your pets' access to certain areas, especially bedrooms.
  - Bathe and brush your pets regularly.
  - Vacuum regularly, and clean the surfaces where your pet spends most of its time.
  - Use air purifiers to reduce airborne allergens.
- Various allergens :
  - Avoid smoking indoors.
  - Choose curtains and blinds that are easy to wash and wash them regularly.
  - Avoid upholstered furniture or choose anti-allergenic coverings.
  - Air the house regularly to renew the air.
  - Use air purifiers to filter out allergens.
- Cockroach and other insects:
  - Keep food in airtight containers.
  - Quickly remove leftovers and crumbs.
  - Use insecticides or cockroach traps if necessary.

- Fix any leaks, as cockroaches are attracted to water.

- Pollen :
    - Keep your windows closed during the pollen season.
    - Use the air conditioning with a clean filter.
    - Shower and change your clothes after spending time outdoors during pollen peaks.

By following these tips and adapting your environment, you can considerably reduce your exposure to household allergens and improve your quality of life.

The importance of healthy indoor air: humidity, ventilation, purifiers

Indoor air quality is crucial to our health and well-being, as we spend a large proportion of our time indoors. Problems with indoor air quality can have a direct impact on health, particularly by exacerbating allergies and respiratory problems. Here's why it's important to maintain healthy indoor air, and how factors such as humidity, ventilation and air purifiers can help:

- Humidity :
    - **Role**: Correctly regulated humidity helps prevent the proliferation of dust mites, mould and certain bacteria.
    - **Risks of excessive humidity**: High humidity levels encourage the growth of mould and dust mites, which are potentially allergenic.
    - **Risks of low humidity**: Air that is too dry can irritate the respiratory tract, cause dry skin and increase vulnerability to viral infections.

- **Recommendation**: It is advisable to maintain relative humidity between 30% and 50%.
- Ventilation :
  - **Role**: Effective ventilation renews indoor air, removing pollutants and reducing allergen levels.
  - **Risks of inadequate ventilation**: This can lead to a build-up of pollutants, such as carbon monoxide, radon, volatile organic compounds (VOCs), tobacco and other allergens.
  - **Recommendation**: Make sure you have adequate ventilation, especially in high-humidity areas such as bathrooms and kitchens. The use of VMC (Ventilation Mécanique Contrôlée) is also recommended.
- Air purifiers :
  - **Role**: They filter the air to remove particles, allergens and sometimes even gases. They can be particularly useful in areas of high pollution or for people suffering from allergies or asthma.
  - **Effect**: Purifiers equipped with HEPA (High Efficiency Particulate Air) filters are effective in removing many particles, including certain allergens such as pet hair, pollen and dust mites.
  - **Recommendation**: If you're thinking of using an air purifier, look for a model suited to the size of your room, and take into account the type and quality of the filter.

Other considerations :
- Take care to reduce the source of pollutants: avoid smoking indoors, use environmentally-friendly household products, avoid construction and decoration materials that emit VOCs, etc.
- Indoor plants can also help improve air quality, although their effectiveness is open to debate.

Maintaining healthy indoor air is crucial to good health. Attention to humidity, ventilation and, where necessary, air purification, can significantly improve the well-being of the occupants of a home or workplace.

The challenges professional environments

Professional environments present specific allergy and immunology challenges. Whether it's an office, a construction site, a factory or a hospital, every workplace has its own risks. Here are some of the main challenges related to allergology and immunology in the workplace:

- **Exposure to specific allergens**: Some jobs expose workers to specific allergens. For example:
    - Bakers can be exposed to flour.
    - Hairdressers can come into contact with chemicals in hair dyes.
    - Healthcare workers can be exposed to latex.
- **Occupational illnesses**: Continuous exposure to certain products or substances can lead to occupational illnesses. For example, asbestos can cause lung disease in construction workers.
- **Indoor air quality**: In buildings that are poorly ventilated or contain building materials that emit volatile organic compounds (VOCs), air quality can be compromised, increasing the risk of allergies and respiratory problems.
- **Stress and the immune system**: Stress at work can affect the immune system, making individuals more vulnerable to infection.
- **Confined environments**: In places such as mines or submarines, exposure to allergens or infectious agents in a confined space can have serious consequences for health.

266

- **Exposure to infectious agents**: Healthcare workers and those working in research laboratories may be exposed to infectious agents, requiring strict prevention protocols.
- **Prevention challenges**: Identifying and reducing occupational risks requires regular workplace assessments, ongoing employee training and the application of safety measures.
- **Recognition and compensation**: When a worker develops a work-related illness or allergy, recognising it as an occupational disease and setting up compensation can be a complex process.

To manage these challenges :
- **Training and education**: Employers must provide regular training on potential hazards and how to avoid them.
- **Regular assessments**: Workplaces must be regularly assessed to identify potential risks.
- **Personal protective equipment**: Provide and require the use of suitable protective equipment, such as masks, gloves and protective clothing.

Preventing and managing allergies and immunological problems in the workplace requires collaboration between employers, employees, health professionals and occupational health experts.

Chapter 32:
EPIDEMIOLOGICAL ASPECTS

Trends and
global allergy statistics

Allergies are among the most common chronic diseases worldwide. In recent decades, there has been a significant increase in the prevalence of different forms of allergy in many parts of the world. Here is an overview of global allergy trends and statistics:

- **Increase in prevalence**: Numerous studies have shown an increase in the prevalence of allergies, particularly in industrialised countries. Allergic diseases such as asthma, allergic rhinitis, atopic dermatitis and food allergies have increased in frequency.
- Food allergies :
    - Food allergies, particularly in children, are on the increase. Common food allergens include peanuts, milk, eggs, soya, wheat, nuts, fish and shellfish.
    - In some countries, such as the United States, up to 8% of children are affected by some form of food allergy.
- **Asthma**: Asthma is one of the most common chronic diseases in children, and also affects a large number of adults. Its prevalence has increased over the last 20 to 30 years.
- Impact of environmental changes :
    - Rising pollution levels and climate change have been associated with an increase in the prevalence of respiratory allergies.

- The phenomenon of the 'hygiene effect', where less exposure to infections in childhood is thought to lead to an increase in allergic responses, has also been suggested as a possible reason.
- Geographical breakdown :
  - Although allergic diseases are common in industrialised   countries, they are also on the increase in developing countries as the latter become more urbanised.
  - There are regional   variations in the prevalence of certain allergies, probably due to environmental, genetic and lifestyle differences.
- **Risk factors**: In addition to genetics, other risk factors include early viral infections, pollution, exposure to certain allergens during childhood and eating habits.
- **Economic costs**: Allergies entail significant costs for healthcare systems due to hospitalisations, medication and loss of productivity. They can also lead to indirect costs, such as missed days at school or work.
- **Awareness and education**: Raising awareness of allergies and their management is essential. Many countries have set up programmes to educate the public and health professionals about allergy prevention and treatment.

Public health is growing on a global scale. A better understanding of the underlying causes and increased awareness can help develop more effective prevention and treatment strategies.

Risk factors and predisposition

Allergies are the result of an exaggerated reaction by the immune system to substances that are generally harmless to most individuals. A number of risk factors and predispositions can increase the likelihood of developing an allergy. Here is an overview of the main risk factors and predispositions associated with allergies:

- Genetic factors :
    - **Family predisposition**: Having parents or siblings who suffer from allergic diseases such as asthma, allergic rhinitis or eczema increases the risk of developing an allergy.
- Environmental factors :
    - **Early exposure**: Early exposure to certain allergens during childhood can increase the risk of developing allergies. However, there is also evidence to suggest that regular exposure to allergens in early childhood may have a protective effect.
    - **Pollution**: Air pollution, particularly indoor pollution caused by factors such as passive smoking, can increase the risk of respiratory allergies.
    - **Climate change**: Changes in the levels of pollens and other airborne allergens due to climate change can affect allergic sensitivity.
    - **Occupational exposure**: Exposure to certain chemicals or materials in the workplace can lead to occupational allergies.
- Health factors :
    - **Early infections**: Certain viral or bacterial infections in early childhood can increase the risk of allergies. For example, early respiratory infections may be associated with an increased risk of asthma.
    - **Mode of birth**: It has been suggested that caesarean section may be associated with a slightly increased risk of allergies, possibly due to differences in microbial exposure at birth.

- Other factors :
  - **Hygiene effect**: The hygiene effect hypothesis suggests that living in an overly clean environment, with less exposure to microbes, may increase the risk of allergies.
  - **Lifestyle**: An unbalanced diet, obesity and lack of physical activity can also contribute to the risk of allergies.
  - **Age**: Although allergies can develop at any age, they are more common in children. However, certain types of allergy, particularly drug allergies, are more common in adults.

It should be noted that allergies are often the result of a complex combination of genetic and environmental factors. Understanding these risk factors and predispositions can help to develop prevention strategies and identify individuals at risk.

Understanding the increase in allergies over time

The increase in allergies over recent decades is a complex and multifactorial phenomenon. Several theories and studies have attempted to explain this growing trend. Here are some of the main reasons and theories that could explain this increase:

- **The hygiene hypothesis**: This theory suggests that living in more sterile environments and having fewer infections during childhood may make the immune system less tolerant and more likely to react to harmless substances. In other words, less exposure to infectious agents in early childhood could predispose us to an increased risk of allergies.

- Environmental change :
  - **Pollution**: Exposure to air pollutants, such as fine particles or vehicle exhaust fumes, can sensitise the respiratory tract and increase the risk of respiratory allergies.
  - **Climate change**: Rising temperatures and CO_2 levels can lead to increased pollen production by certain plants, extending the pollen season.
- Dietary factors :
  - **Western diet**: A diet high in saturated fats and sugar and low in fibre could play a role in the increase in allergies.
  - **Late introduction of allergenic foods**: In the past, recommendations often suggested delaying the introduction of potentially allergenic foods. However, more recent studies suggest that early introduction of these foods may actually reduce the risk of allergies.
- **Use of antibiotics**: Taking antibiotics, especially in the first few years of life, can disrupt the intestinal microbiota, which could increase the risk of allergies.
- **Indoor living**: Spending more time indoors, with reduced ventilation and increased exposure to indoor allergens such as house dust mites, can increase the risk of allergies.
- **Genetic factors**: Although genes have not changed as rapidly as the incidence of allergies, it is possible that certain genetic factors interact with the environmental factors mentioned above to increase the risk of allergies.
- **Urbanisation**: Living in an urban environment, with reduced exposure to the microbial diversity found in rural environments, could increase the risk of allergies.

- **Social pressure and diagnosis**: Greater awareness of allergies and improved access to care can lead to more frequent diagnosis.

It is important to note that the increase in allergies is probably due to a combination of several of these factors. In addition, the incidence of allergies can vary between regions and populations. Research continues to be carried out to fully understand the causes of this increase and to develop effective prevention strategies.

Importance
epidemiological surveillance

Epidemiological surveillance is a crucial element of public health. It refers to the regular collection, analysis, interpretation and dissemination of health-related information, with the aim of preventing and controlling disease. Here's why it's so important:

- **Early detection of epidemics**: Surveillance enables the early detection of new epidemics or the resurgence of known diseases. This early detection facilitates rapid intervention, thereby limiting the spread of the disease.
- **Understanding trends and patterns**: By tracking the evolution of diseases over time, epidemiological surveillance makes it possible to identify trends, at-risk groups, the geographical areas affected and the seasons of predilection for certain diseases.
- **Evaluation of interventions**: Surveillance provides data to assess the effectiveness of interventions, whether they be vaccination campaigns, health education or any other programme.
- **Allocation of resources**: Thanks to surveillance, public health officials can allocate resources where

they are most needed, based on the prevalence or incidence of disease.

- **Research**: Epidemiological data feeds into research, helping to identify the causes of disease, risk factors and opportunities for intervention.
- **Emergency preparedness and response**: In the event of an epidemic or pandemic, it is essential to have up-to-date, accurate data so that the appropriate responses can be implemented.
- **Health policy development**: Decision-makers rely on surveillance data to develop, adapt or evaluate public health policies and strategies.
- **Public education**: Surveillance data can be used to educate the public about health risks, modes of disease transmission and preventive measures.
- **International liaison**: In an increasingly interconnected world, epidemiological surveillance enables information to be shared between countries, making it easier to coordinate responses to cross-border threats.
- **Identifying new threats**: In addition to known diseases, epidemiological surveillance can help detect the emergence of new pathologies or new strains of existing diseases.

When properly conducted, epidemiological surveillance plays a key role in protecting the health of populations. It requires rigorous data collection, statistical analysis, judicious interpretation and effective communication to achieve its full potential.

Chapter 33:
INTERPROFESSIONAL COLLABORATION

Teamwork with doctors, pharmacists and dieticians

Multidisciplinary teamwork, particularly in healthcare, is fundamental to providing comprehensive, coordinated care for patients. Each professional brings specific skills and a particular vision of care. Here are some key points about teamwork with doctors, pharmacists, dieticians and other healthcare professionals:

- Complementary skills :
    - **Doctors**: Diagnose, prescribe treatment and coordinate care.
    - **Pharmacists**: Advise on medicines, their side effects and interactions, and ensure correct dispensing.
    - **Dieticians**: Offer nutritional advice tailored to the patient's pathology or condition.
    - **Nurses**: They are responsible for day-to-day monitoring, administering treatment and therapeutic education, and are often the first point of contact for patients.
- **Fluid communication**: Open and respectful communication is essential for sharing information, asking questions, clarifying doubts and discussing the best treatment plans for the patient.
- **Regular meetings**: These meetings are used to discuss complex cases, adjust treatments and ensure that every member of the team is on the same wavelength.

- **Focus on the patient**: The main objective is always the patient's well-being. Each professional must put egos and differences aside to focus on what is best for the patient.
- **Ongoing training**: Constantly evolving medical knowledge means that every member of the team needs to keep up to date. This also helps us to better understand and respect the role of each professional.
- **Educational role**: In addition to direct care, the team also has an educational role. Whether it's teaching patients how to manage their disease, providing information on the side effects of medication or giving appropriate dietary advice.
- **Care coordination**: Ensuring a smooth transition between the different levels of care (hospitalisation, home care, specialist consultations) is crucial to continuity of care.
- **Referrals**: Depending on the patient's needs, the team may refer them to other specialists or services (psychology, physiotherapy, etc.).
- **Documentation and information sharing**: Keeping records that are up to date and accessible to all team members helps to ensure consistent care.
- **Mutual respect**: Each member of the team must value and respect the skills and opinions of others, even when they disagree.

The multidisciplinary approach is now recognised as one of the most effective ways of ensuring comprehensive, personalised care for patients. It does, however, require a commitment to collaboration, communication and ongoing training on the part of all its members.

The importance of communication and care coordination

Communication and care coordination are fundamental in the healthcare sector to ensure optimal patient care. Not only do they improve clinical outcomes, they also strengthen the patient-healthcare professional relationship, optimise resources and prevent medical errors. Here's why these two elements are of vital importance:

- Patient Safety :
    - Effective communication reduces the risk of medical errors, omissions or duplication of prescriptions and treatments.
    - It ensures that every professional involved in a patient's care is informed about the procedures, allergies, contraindications and medical history.
- Continuity   of care :
    - Coordination ensures a seamless transition between the different levels and players involved in care (hospital, clinic, home care, GP, specialists, etc.).
    - It avoids treatment interruptions and ensures that patients receive consistent care at every stage of their medical journey.

- Optimising Resources :
    - Avoids redundant tests or procedures, saving time and money.
    - Ensures that medical   resources are used efficiently.
- Patient satisfaction :
    - Good communication and coordination boost patients' confidence in healthcare professionals.

- They ensure that the patient is well informed, which can reduce anxiety and encourage adherence to treatment.
- Shared Decision :
  - Communication encourages shared decision-making between the patient and healthcare professionals, enabling care to be tailored to the patient's needs and wishes.
- Chronic Disease Management :
  - Coordination is essential for patients suffering from chronic illnesses requiring the intervention of multiple healthcare professionals.
- Strengthening the medical team :
  - Open and respectful communication between professionals strengthens team cohesion, enables knowledge to be shared and improves care.
- Emergency Management :
  - In critical situations, clear and rapid communication is essential if we are to act effectively and safely.
- Education and Understanding :
  - Good communication ensures that patients understand their illness, their treatment and the measures they need to take to maintain their health.
- Respect and Dignity:
  - By communicating empathetically and coordinating care, healthcare professionals show respect for the patient, thereby strengthening the therapeutic relationship.

Communication and care coordination are the cornerstones of modern, patient-centred medicine. Implementing them requires training, commitment and appropriate tools (such as electronic medical records), but the benefits for patients and the healthcare system in general are immense.

Case studies: success stories inter-professional collaboration

Interprofessional collaboration in healthcare is essential for comprehensive, optimal patient care. Here are a few case studies illustrating notable successes thanks to these collaborations:

1. Chronic Pain Management :

Situation: A patient suffering from chronic pain linked to osteoarthritis was being treated by his general practitioner. Despite several medications, the pain persisted, affecting his quality of life.

Intervention: A team comprising a rheumatologist, a physiotherapist, a psychologist and a pharmacist worked together to provide comprehensive care.

Result: Thanks to a combined approach (adjustment of medication, physical therapy and stress management strategies), the patient's pain was significantly reduced.

2. Diabetes management :

Situation: A diabetic patient was having difficulty controlling her blood sugar levels despite taking her medication.

Intervention: A team including an endocrinologist, a dietician, a nurse specialising in diabetes and a chiropodist looked into her case.

Result: The patient benefited from a suitable diet, education on self-monitoring of blood sugar levels, and treatment for her feet (at risk of ulcers). Her diabetes is now well controlled.

3. Eating Disorders in Adolescents :

Situation: An adolescent girl was suffering from severe anorexia nervosa.

Intervention: A team comprising a paediatrician, a psychiatrist, a nutritionist and a psychologist worked together to provide comprehensive care.

Result: The teenager received medical, nutritional and psychological support, and gradually regained her weight while treating the underlying causes of her disorder.

4. Stroke rehabilitation :

Situation: A patient has suffered a stroke with partial paralysis of the right side.

Intervention: A team comprising a neurologist, a physiotherapist, an occupational therapist and a speech therapist looked after the patient.

Result: After several months of integrated and interprofessional rehabilitation, the patient recovered a large part of his motor functions and learned to speak properly again.

5. Dementia Management :

Situation: An elderly patient has been diagnosed with incipient dementia.

Intervention: A team comprising a geriatrician, a neurologist, a specialist geriatric nurse, a psychologist and a social worker drew up a care plan.

Result: Thanks to appropriate medical monitoring, cognitive stimulation and social support, the progression of the disease was slowed down, and the patient was able to stay at home for longer than expected.

These case studies illustrate the importance of interprofessional collaboration. When each professional contributes his or her specific expertise, patient care is more comprehensive, more effective and better adapted to individual needs.

Challenges and best practice for integrated care

Integrated care is a model of care that aims to provide a coordinated and comprehensive response to a person's health needs. This approach requires close collaboration between different healthcare professionals and other stakeholders. While this model has many advantages, such as improving the quality of care and reducing costs, it also presents challenges.

Challenges of integrated care :
- **Interprofessional communication**: Clear and effective communication between professionals is essential, but it can be complicated by language barriers, different levels of training or different specialisations.
- **Technological integration**: The use of electronic medical records and other technologies may vary from one professional to another, making coordination difficult.
- **Training and education**: Not all the professionals involved may have the necessary training to work in an integrated setting.
- **Resistance to change**: Some professionals may be reluctant to adopt a new model of care for fear of losing their professional autonomy.
- **Financial issues**: Financing integrated care can be complex, particularly in multi-payer healthcare systems.

Best practices for effective integrated care :
- **Interprofessional training**: training professionals to work as part of a team, to understand the roles of others and to communicate effectively.
- **Consistent technological tools**: Adopt common technological platforms, such as electronic medical

records, which enable transparent, real-time communication.

- **Established care protocols**: Establish clear protocols for patient care, ensuring that they are adapted to the specific needs of each patient.
- **Coordination centres**: create specific centres or teams responsible for coordinating care, ensuring communication between professionals and monitoring care plans.
- **Ongoing evaluation**: Put in place evaluation and feedback mechanisms to regularly assess the effectiveness of integrated care and identify areas for improvement.
- **Patient Engagement**: Including patients and their families in the decision-making process, and ensuring that they are informed and educated about their condition and care plan.
- **Appropriate funding**: Work with payers to establish funding models that support and encourage integrated care.

Integrated care, when implemented effectively, has the potential to improve the quality of care, increase patient and healthcare professional satisfaction, and reduce costs. A collaborative approach, supported by appropriate training, appropriate technology and adequate funding, is essential to overcome the challenges and realise the full potential of this model.

Chapter 34:
FUTURE DEVELOPMENTS
IN ALLERGOLOGY
AND IMMUNOLOGY

New research and treatments

The fields of allergology and immunology are constantly evolving, with major advances in our understanding of the underlying mechanisms and the development of innovative treatments. Here's a look at some of the promising new research and treatments:

- **Monoclonal Antibody Biology**: These drugs, specifically designed to target certain proteins involved in allergic and immune reactions, offer treatment options for conditions such as severe asthma, atopic dermatitis and other severe allergies.
- **Gene therapy**: Progress has been made in the treatment of primary immunodeficiency disorders thanks to gene therapy. These techniques aim to correct the genetic defect that causes the disease.
- **Microbiome and allergies**: Research is exploring how imbalances in gut bacteria (the microbiome) can influence the development of allergies. Probiotics and other interventions to restore a healthy microbiome are being studied to prevent or treat allergies.
- **Rapid desensitisation**: Accelerated protocols for desensitisation to allergens such as food or insect venoms are being developed. These techniques enable desensitisation to take place in a few hours rather than several months.

- **Vaccines for allergies**: Vaccines are being studied to treat or prevent certain allergies, particularly food allergies.
- **Treatment of food allergies**: New treatments, such as immunotherapy skin patches and oral therapies, are being tested to treat food allergies such as peanut allergy.
- **Stem Cell Therapies**: Stem cells may have the potential to regenerate or repair damaged tissue in certain immunological diseases.
- **Technological approaches**: The adoption of telemedicine, mobile applications and monitoring devices is enabling better monitoring of allergic and immunocompromised patients.
- **Treatment of Chronic Urticaria**: New therapeutic targets and drugs are being developed to treat chronic urticaria, a condition which can be disabling for some patients.
- **Biomarker Identification**: Research into biomarkers to predict the severity, prognosis and response to treatment of allergic and immunological diseases.

These advances are the fruit of fundamental research, clinical trials and interdisciplinary collaboration. While some of these treatments are already available, others are still under study. However, these advances offer the hope of a better quality of life for patients suffering from allergic and immunological diseases.

Developments in diagnostic techniques

Diagnostic techniques in allergology and immunology have evolved considerably over the last few decades. Improvements in these techniques allow more precise identification of the allergens responsible for symptoms and a better understanding of the underlying immunological mechanisms. Here is an overview of these developments:

- Skin tests :
  - **Prick Tests**: Although the basic technique remains similar, the range of allergens tested has broadened. What's more, improved devices allow for greater standardisation of application.
  - **Intradermal tests**: Used mainly for allergens to which prick tests are less sensitive.
- Specific IgE assay :
  - Initially, tests were limited to measuring total IgE. Nowadays, IgE antibodies specific to different allergens are measured, providing greater precision in identifying the allergen responsible.
  - **ImmunoCAP technology**: Enables the determination of specific IgE antibodies for a wide range of allergens.
- Provocation tests :
  - Although they are older, they remain the benchmark for diagnosing certain allergies, particularly food allergies. Techniques and protocols have been refined to reduce risks.
- Cytophoniqutest (Basophil Activation Test) :
  - Measures the reaction of basophils (a type of white blood cell) in the presence of an allergen. This technique is particularly useful in cases where skin tests and specific IgE are inconclusive.
- Patch Testing :
  - Used to identify allergens responsible for contact dermatitis. The range of substances tested has expanded with the recognition of new allergens.

- Microarray technology :
  - These chips can detect thousands of allergens simultaneously from a single sample, enabling a detailed assessment of a patient's allergy profile.
- Imaging techniques :
  - Particularly in cases of asthma or other allergy-related lung conditions. Developments in imaging techniques, such as computed tomography (CT) and magnetic resonance imaging (MRI), offer more precise images of inflammation and other changes in the lungs.
- Immune Function Assessment :
  - Advanced tests, such as lymphocyte subpopulation assays, lymphoproliferative response measurements and the detection of specific proteins, enable primary and secondary immune deficiencies to be diagnosed and monitored.

With these advances, the accuracy and efficiency of the diagnosis of allergies and immunological disorders have greatly improved, leading to more appropriate treatment plans and a better quality of life for patients.

Future challenges for nurses

The role of the allergology nurse, as in other areas of healthcare, is constantly evolving. Several challenges await these professionals in the future:

- Increasing complexity of care :
  - With technological and therapeutic advances, patient care is becoming increasingly complex. Nurses need to keep abreast of the latest advances to provide optimum care.

- Technology integration :
    - Telemedicine, electronic medical records, remote monitoring devices, etc. all require ongoing training and adaptation.
- Management of Multimorbid Patients :
    - Many allergy patients have other medical conditions. Managing these co-morbidities requires a holistic approach and coordinated care.
- Patient Education :
    - With the increase in allergic diseases, education of patients and their families is becoming crucial. This includes teaching prevention, symptom recognition and crisis management.
- Managing Stress and Burnout :
    - The healthcare environment is demanding, and the risk of burnout is high. Finding strategies to manage stress and maintain work-life balance is crucial.
- Changes to the regulatory framework :
    - Laws and regulations can change, affecting nurses' practice. Keeping abreast of and adapting to these changes is a constant challenge.
- Interprofessional collaboration :
    - Working in a team with other healthcare professionals (doctors, pharmacists, dieticians, etc.) requires effective communication and coordination.
- Cultural diversity :
    - Nurses may have to deal with patients from different cultural backgrounds and must therefore be trained in cultural competence in order to provide respectful and appropriate care.

- Antimicrobial resistance:
    - With drug resistance on the   r i s e ,
      particularly in immunocompromised patients,
      nurses need to be vigilant and well-informed
      about best practice.
- Ethical Challenges :
    - Nurses may be faced with ethical dilemmas,
      such as refusing treatment, end-of-life
      decisions or genetic issues.
- The need for nursing research :
    - Contributing to research and scientific evidence
      in the field of allergology nursing is essential for
      the advancement of the profession.

In the face of these challenges, continuing education,
research, professional support and effective collaboration
are essential to enable nurses to offer the best possible
care to their patients.

Chapter 35:
CONCLUSION AND OUTLOOK

The central role of the nurse in Allergology and Immunology

The Allergy and Immunology nurse occupies a unique and essential position within the medical team. She is often the first point of contact for patients experiencing symptoms of allergy or immune disorders, acting as a bridge between them and the complex world of specialist medicine. Her role extends far beyond basic clinical interventions; she is also an educator, counsellor, researcher and patient advocate.

In the hustle and bustle of the medical consultation, the nurse is the reassuring figure who takes the time to listen and understand patients' concerns. She translates medical jargon into understandable terms, helping patients to decode their symptoms, diagnoses and treatment options. This communication is essential if patients are to feel involved, listened to and understood in their care.

Nurses also play a vital educational role. In the field of allergology, for example, she instructs patients on how to avoid allergens, teaches them to recognise the signs of a severe allergic reaction and guides them on the correct use of treatments such as epinephrine auto-injectors. For patients with immune deficiencies, it offers advice on how to reduce the risk of infections and ensure that their lives are as normal and fulfilling as possible.

Nurses are also at the forefront of clinical research. They are often involved in the implementation and monitoring of clinical trials, contributing to the advancement of new therapies and treatment strategies. This role as researcher reinforces the importance of continuing education, as nurses need to keep up to date with the latest discoveries and innovations.

Finally, as an advocate, the nurse fights for the rights of her patients, ensuring that they receive appropriate care, are treated with dignity and respect, and have access to the necessary resources. She advocates greater awareness of allergies and immune deficiencies, highlighting the need for better recognition, early diagnosis and effective treatment.

In short, the allergy and immunology nurse is not simply a person who carries out medical orders; she is a central pillar of the medical team. Thanks to her versatility, dedication and proximity to patients, she ensures that they receive holistic, informed and caring care.

The importance of ongoing training

Continuing education is a fundamental element in the career of any healthcare professional, and this is particularly true for nurses. In a world where medical knowledge
In a world where health care is evolving at a frenetic pace and medical technology is constantly advancing, the need to keep up to date has never been more crucial.

Firstly, continuing education ensures that nurses can provide the best possible care to their patients. Emerging therapies, new diagnostic techniques and advances in patient management are constantly changing the way care is delivered. Without regular updating of knowledge, it would be easy for a professional to rely on outdated methods, which may not be the most beneficial for the patient.

Secondly, it helps to reinforce professional confidence. A nurse who is well informed about the latest practices is more likely to feel competent in her role. This confidence translates not only into better patient care, but also into better interaction with other members of the care team.

Continuing education is also essential for career progression. In many healthcare systems around the world, progression up the professional hierarchy or specialisation often requires additional qualifications or certifications that can only be obtained through continuing education. In addition, it opens doors to opportunities such as teaching, research or advisory roles.

Furthermore, in an increasingly globalised world, continuing education enables nurses to understand international practices, emerging diseases and global protocols. This can be particularly relevant for nurses who work in tourist areas, cosmopolitan cities, or who are considering working abroad.

Finally, beyond the practical benefits, there is an intrinsic benefit to learning itself. Curiosity, a desire to know more and to improve, are traits inherent in many healthcare professionals. Continuing education feeds this thirst for knowledge, offering intellectual stimulation and personal satisfaction.

Continuing education is more than just an obligation or a chore. It's an opportunity for nurses to enhance their skills, improve their practice and ensure that they are always providing the best possible care for their patients. In a field as vital and dynamic as healthcare, stagnation is simply not an option.

Encourage
the new generation of nurses

In an increasingly complex and specialised world, the role of the nurse has become essential to the smooth running of healthcare systems. Encouraging the next generation of nurses is therefore of paramount importance. Here's how we can inspire and support the next wave of dedicated carers:

- **Promoting the profession**: It is vital to highlight the successes and significant contributions of nurses in the healthcare sector. Sharing inspiring stories and testimonials can motivate young people to consider a career in nursing.
- **Mentoring**: Experienced nurses should be encouraged to become mentors to new recruits, offering advice, support and a valuable perspective on the profession.
- **Learning opportunities**: Continuing education programmes, workshops and seminars should be made available to young nurses to help them develop their skills and keep abreast of the latest medical advances.
- **Encouraging diversity**: It is crucial to encourage people from different backgrounds to join the nursing profession, thereby enriching the diversity of experience and perspectives within the profession.
- **Promoting nursing research**: Supporting and promoting research carried out by nurses recognises their crucial role not only as care providers, but also as researchers.
- **Offering varied career opportunities**: It is essential to show young nurses that there are a multitude of possible career paths, whether they specialise in specific areas, work abroad or go into research or teaching.

- **Ensuring a healthy working environment**: A positive working environment, where nurses' well-being and mental health are taken into account, will attract more young people to the profession.
- **Commitment to education**: Educational institutions must continue to innovate in their nursing education programmes, ensuring that they are relevant, up-to-date and patient-centred.
- **Networking**: Encourage young nurses to join professional associations where they can meet other professionals, exchange experience and knowledge, and benefit from valuable resources.
- **Recognition and rewards**: Recognition and reward programmes can motivate nurses, showing that their efforts and dedication are appreciated.

The new generation of nurses is the promise of a robust and resilient healthcare system for the future. By supporting them, valuing them and investing in their education and well-being, we will ensure not only quality care for patients, but also sustainability and innovation in nursing.